NON-HODGKIN LYMPHOMA COOKBOOK

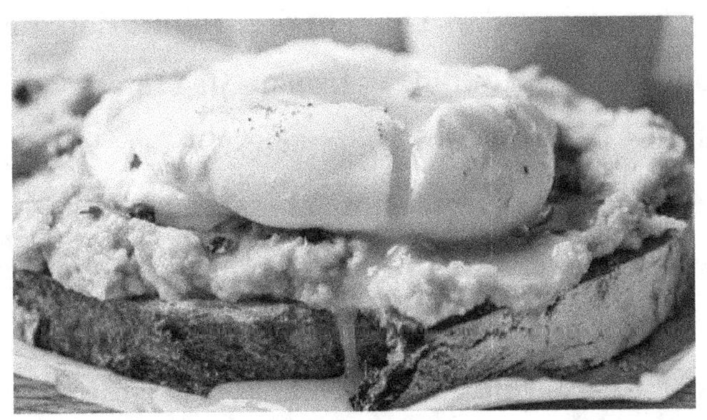

Essential Recipes for Recovery with Cancer-Fighting Foods Featuring Anti-Inflammatory Ingredients for Optimal Wellness and Resilience

LENA R. FOSTER

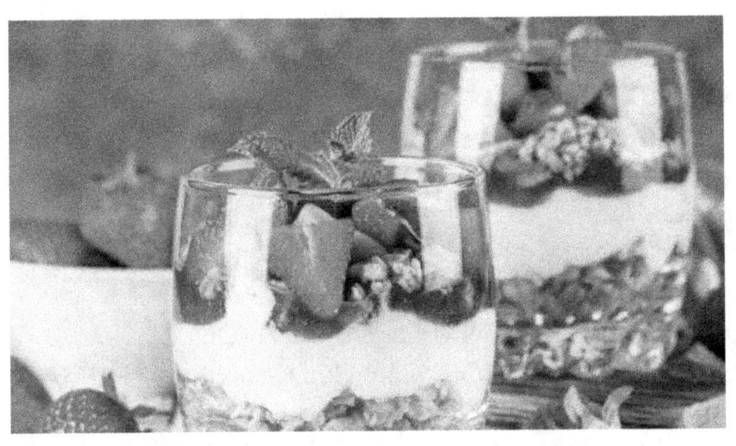

NON-HODGKIN LYMPHOMA COOKBOOK

Table of Contents

INTRODUCTION

Lena's struggle with Non-Hodgkin Lymphoma was difficult, but her drive to reclaim control of her health led her to a unique solution: a Non-Hodgkin Lymphoma Cookbook. Frustrated with traditional therapy, Lena began to investigate the possible advantages of a personalized diet.

The cookbook, created by oncology and nutrition specialists, supplied Lena with recipes including anti-inflammatory foods and immune-boosting elements. Lena followed this culinary road map, eating nutritious grains, lean meats, and plenty of fruits and vegetables.

Lena saw a gradual improvement in her energy levels and general well-being. She shared her story with a supportive network of others suffering similar issues, motivating them to live better lives.

Through this culinary transformation, Lena did not only healed her Non-Hodgkin Lymphoma but also gave her a renewed respect for the therapeutic potential of nutritional foods. Her path became a beacon of hope for others navigating the difficulties of cancer, demonstrating that the correct ingredients in the kitchen may be just as effective as any medication.

Lena's narrative demonstrated the enormous influence of a well-crafted cookbook on her quest to restore a healthy and vibrant lifestyle.

Welcome to this Non-Hodgkin Lymphoma Cookbook, a culinary guide created to help people overcome Non-Hodgkin Lymphoma via the transformational power of nutrition. These pages provide a carefully chosen selection of recipes designed to promote general well-being, improve immunological function, and establish a good link between food and health.

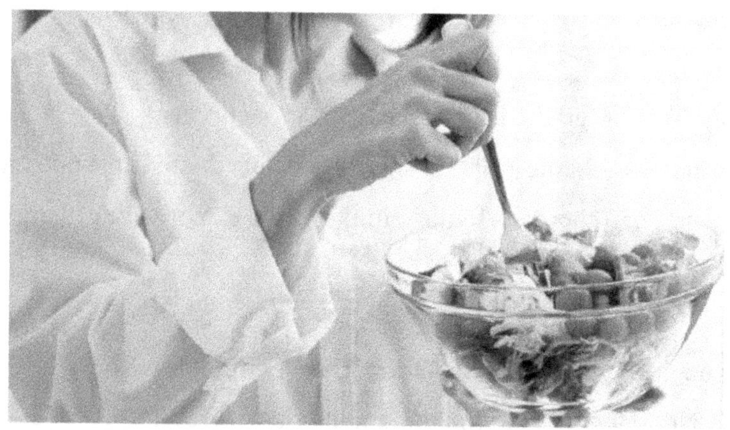

HOW THIS COOKBOOK CAN HELP

1. Customized Nutrition: Offers recipes tailored to unique dietary needs during treatment, ensuring individuals receive the right nutrients to support their health.

2. Treatment Challenge Management: Includes easy-to-follow recipes to combat side effects like nausea and taste changes, ensuring that every meal is both fun and healthy.

3. Immune Function Boost: Recipes high in vitamins, minerals, and antioxidants to strengthen the immune system, which is essential during Non-Hodgkin Lymphoma therapy.

4. Diverse and Enjoyable Meals: Say good-bye to monotony! This cookbook promotes a varied diet to stick to nutritional objectives.

5. Practical Living Tips: Includes ideas for grocery shopping and meal preparation. It's a complete guide to smoothly incorporating healthy meals into your daily routine, promoting overall well-being throughout treatment.

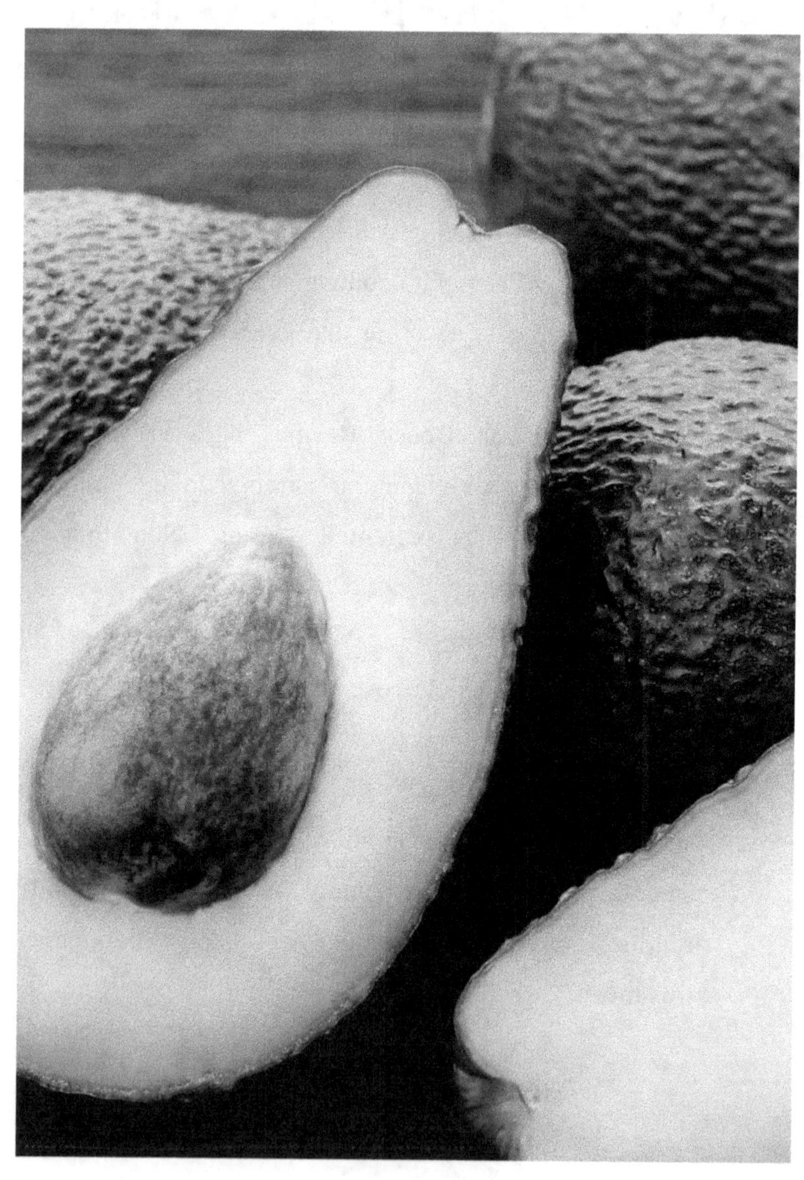

CHAPTER 1: UNDERSTANDING NON-HODGKIN LYMPHOMA

Non-Hodgkin lymphoma (NHL) is a malignancy that develops in the lymphatic system, which is an essential component of the immune system. Unlike Hodgkin lymphoma, NHL has several subtypes, making it a heterogeneous collection of blood malignancies.

CAUSES AND RISK FACTORS

The precise cause of NHL is unknown, however some risk factors enhance susceptibility. These include age, with the incidence increasing with age, immunodeficiency conditions, chemical exposure, and a family history of lymphoma.

TYPES OF NON-HODGKIN LYMPHOMA

Non-Hodgkin Lymphoma is classified into several subtypes depending on the afflicted lymphocyte type (B-cells or T-cells) and growth pattern. Diffuse large B-cell lymphoma, follicular lymphoma, and mantle cell lymphoma are three common subtypes, each with its own set of features and therapeutic options.

SYMPTOMS

Symptoms of NHL may include swollen lymph nodes, fever, night sweats, weight loss, exhaustion, and abdominal discomfort. A timely diagnosis is critical for successful treatment.

DIAGNOSIS

NHL is diagnosed using a combination of medical history, physical examination, imaging tests (CT scans, MRI), and a biopsy of lymph node tissue under a microscope. This thorough method aids in the determination of the disease's subtype and severity.

STAGING

NHL is staged to determine its spread and inform treatment recommendations. The stages range from I-IV. Stage I and II NHL are called early stages (limited) while III and IV NHL are called advanced Lymphoma (widespread). Accurate staging is essential in developing an effective treatment approach.

TREATMENT OPTIONS

Treatment options for NHL differ according to subtype, stage, and specific patient variables. Common treatments include chemotherapy, immunotherapy, radiation therapy, and stem cell transplantation. Targeted medicines that target particular molecular characteristics of cancer cells are now emerging as viable possibilities.

PROGNOSIS

NHL prognosis varies according to subtype, stage, and therapy response. While some subtypes have positive results, others may provide issues. Regular follow-ups and monitoring are essential for long-term treatment.

SUPPORT AND COPING

Living with the NHL may be emotionally difficult. Support groups, counseling, and building a strong support network may help you cope with the physical and emotional elements of the condition.

IMPORTANCE OF NUTRITION DURING TREATMENT

Nutrition is critical in supporting those receiving medical treatment, especially cancer therapy. Maintaining healthy nutrition during treatments such as chemotherapy, radiation, or surgery is vital for various reasons:

1. Energy and Strength: Cancer treatments may cause exhaustion and decreased energy levels. Adequate diet supplies critical nutrients to sustain energy, assisting patients in maintaining strength throughout the difficult stages of therapy.

2. Immune System Support: Proper diet is essential for a healthy immune system. Cancer therapies may damage the immune system, therefore it is important to eat a well-balanced diet rich in vitamins, minerals, and antioxidants to boost immune function and lower the risk of infection.

3. Tissue Repair and Healing: Surgery and cancer treatments may cause tissue damage. Protein, zinc, and vitamins help in tissue regeneration and healing, allowing the body to recover more efficiently.

4. Managing Side Effects: Cancer therapies can cause nausea, appetite loss, and taste abnormalities. Individualizing the diet to patients' tastes and tolerances may help control these adverse effects while also ensuring they get enough nutrients.

5. Weight Maintenance: Keeping a healthy weight is essential throughout cancer therapy. Proper eating helps to avoid excessive weight loss, which may affect treatment tolerance and general well-being. On the other hand, it may help prevent harmful weight gain in situations when inactivity is common.

6. Blood Cell Production: Cancer therapies, especially chemotherapy, may impact blood cell formation. Consuming meals high in iron, folate, and vitamin B12 helps to produce red blood cells, reducing anemia and weariness.

7. Digestive Health: Cancer therapies may cause digestive difficulties, including diarrhea and constipation. A well-balanced diet that includes fiber-rich foods promotes digestive health and may help reduce some of these issues.

8. Psychological Well-being: Eating a nutritious dict may improve a patient's psychological well-being. Good diet is connected to mood and cognitive performance, which helps to maintain a feeling of well-being throughout difficult times.

9. Individualized Nutrition Plans: Each patient has distinct nutritional requirements. Developing a tailored nutrition plan ensures that individuals obtain the nutrients required for their condition and treatment.

10. Long-term Health: Developing appropriate dietary habits throughout cancer treatment promotes long-term health. Maintaining a healthy diet after treatment may help with healing, lower the chance of cancer recurrence, and improve general health.

FOODS TO EAT AND FOODS TO AVOID

FOODS TO EAT

1. Lean Proteins: Include lean protein sources such chicken, fish, tofu, and lentils. These supply the essential amino acids required for tissue repair and immunological function.

2. Colorful Fruits and Vegetables: Eat a range of colorful fruits and vegetables high in antioxidants, vitamins, and minerals. These improve general health and counteract oxidative stress after non-Hodgkin lymphoma therapy.

3. Whole Grains: Choose whole grains, including brown rice, quinoa, and whole wheat bread. They include complex carbs that give long-term energy and fiber that promotes digestive health.

4. Healthy Fats: Consume healthy fats, such avocados, nuts, seeds, and olive oil. These fats improve general health and may help people lose weight.

5. Dairy or Dairy Alternatives: Choose low-fat dairy or dairy substitutes with calcium and vitamin D. These nutrients are essential for bone health, particularly during cancer therapy.

6. Hydrating Beverages: Stay hydrated with water, herbal teas, and clear broths. Proper hydration helps to manage adverse effects such as nausea while also supporting general physiological processes.

7. Small, Frequent Meals: Eat modest, frequent meals to control hunger and decrease nausea. This method helps to keep energy levels stable throughout the day.

FOODS TO AVOID

1. Processed Foods: Reduce consumption of processed and packaged foods rich in preservatives, additives, and salt. These may increase inflammation and may not give enough nutrients.

2. Sugary Foods and Beverages: Limit sugary meals and drinks, since they may lead to weight gain and severely damage health. Use natural sweeteners in moderation.

3. Reduce Consumption of High-Fat and Fried Foods: These foods are difficult to digest and may cause digestive pain.

4. Alcohol: Limit or prevent alcohol use since it may interact with drugs and harm the liver, particularly during cancer treatment.

5. Caffeine: Consume moderately to avoid dehydration. If necessary, choose herbal teas or decaffeinated choices.

SHOPPING LIST FOR NON-HODGKIN LYMPHOMA

Fruits

- Berries (blueberries, strawberries)
- Citrus fruits (oranges, grapefruits)
- Apples
- Bananas

Vegetables

- Leafy greens (spinach, kale)
- Cruciferous vegetables (broccoli, cauliflower)
- Carrots
- Bell peppers

Whole Grains

- Quinoa
- Brown rice
- Whole wheat pasta
- Oats

Lean Proteins

- Skinless chicken breast
- Turkey

- Fish (salmon, mackerel)
- Tofu

Dairy or Dairy Alternatives

- Low-fat or Greek yogurt
- Skim milk or almond milk

Healthy Fats

- Avocados
- Nuts (almonds, walnuts)
- Olive oil

Beans and Legumes

- Chickpeas
- Lentils
- Black beans

Hydration

- Water
- Herbal teas

Herbs and Spices

- Turmeric
- Ginger

- Garlic

- Basil

- Cilantro

Snacks

- Hummus

- Whole grain crackers

- Nut butter

TIPS FOR MAINTAINING A HEALTHY DIET

Eating healthy is critical for those coping with Non-Hodgkin Lymphoma. Proper eating can help manage symptoms and promote overall well-being.

Here are some tips from this Non-Hodgkin Lymphoma Cookbook to help you keep a healthy diet:

1. Prioritize Nutrient-Dense Foods: Focus on foods high in important nutrients, such as fruits, vegetables, whole grains, lean meats, and healthy fats. These meals give the body the energy and nourishment it requires to function properly.

2. Stay Hydrated: Adequate hydration is essential for general health. Drink enough water throughout the day to maintain appropriate body processes and aid digestion. Herbal teas and infused water can provide diversity while maintaining hydration levels.

3. Select Anti-inflammatory Foods: Include anti-inflammatory foods to help control inflammation caused by Non-Hodgkin Lymphoma. Include turmeric, ginger, garlic, and omega-3 fatty acids from foods such as salmon and flaxseeds.

4. Go for Lean Proteins: Choose lean proteins such as skinless chicken, fish, tofu, and lentils. Protein is required to maintain muscle mass and assist the immune system throughout therapy.

5. Moderate Portion Sizes: To avoid overeating, keep your portion proportions in check. Eating smaller, more often meals throughout the day may be simpler to handle, especially if the medication has decreased your appetite.

6. Mindful Eating: Savor each meal while paying attention to hunger and fullness indicators. This might help you appreciate your meals more and avoid overeating.

7. Include Fiber-Rich foods: To promote digestive health, eat fiber-rich meals such as whole grains, fruits, and vegetables. Fiber can also assist with constipation, which is a typical side effect of several medications.

8. Limit Processed Foods: Reduce consumption of processed and high-sugar foods. These can cause inflammation and may not contain the nutrients required for healthy health.

9. Customize for Individual Needs: Everyone's dietary requirements are unique. Consult a healthcare practitioner or nutritionist to customize the diet depending on your own preferences, treatment side effects, and unique health concerns.

10. Experiment with Flavorful Herbs & Spices: Use fragrant herbs and spices such as basil, cilantro, and rosemary to enhance the taste of your food. Experimenting with different spices may make food more attractive, especially if taste preferences change.

CHAPTER 2: 30-DAY MEAL PLAN

DAY 1

BREAKFAST: Quinoa Breakfast Bowl

LUNCH: Quinoa Salad with Roasted Vegetables

SNACK: Hummus and Veggie Snack Platter

DINNER: Baked Chicken Breast with Sweet Potato and Asparagus

DAY 2

BREAKFAST: Avocado Toast with Poached Egg

LUNCH: Mediterranean Chickpea Bowl

SNACK: Apple Almond Energy Bites

DINNER: Lemon Garlic Shrimp Stir-Fry with Broccoli and Brown Rice

DAY 3

BREAKFAST: Greek Yogurt Parfait

LUNCH: Turkey and Quinoa Stuffed Bell Peppers

SNACK: Edamame and Avocado Salsa

DINNER: Vegetarian Lentil and Spinach Stuffed Bell Peppers

DAY 4

BREAKFAST: Oatmeal Banana Pancakes

LUNCH: Salmon and Vegetable Stir-Fry

SNACK: Roasted Chickpeas with Turmeric and Cumin

DINNER: Sesame Ginger Tofu Stir-Fry

DAY 5

BREAKFAST: Spinach and Feta Egg Muffins

LUNCH: Vegetarian Lentil and Vegetable Soup

SNACK: Spinach and Feta Stuffed Mushrooms

DINNER: Salmon and Quinoa Salad with Lemon Dill Dressing

DAY 6

BREAKFAST: Chia Seed Pudding with Berries

LUNCH: Quinoa and Chickpea Salad Bowl

SNACK: Almond Butter and Banana Rice Cakes

DINNER: Lemon Herb Baked Cod with Roasted Vegetables

DAY 7

BREAKFAST: Sweet Potato and Kale Breakfast Hash

LUNCH: Turkey and Vegetable Lettuce Wraps

SNACK: Cucumber Hummus Bites

DINNER: Vegetarian Lentil Curry with Quinoa

DAY 8

BREAKFAST: Cottage Cheese and Fruit Bowl

LUNCH: Sweet Potato and Black Bean Quinoa Bowl

SNACK: Zucchini and Walnut Muffins

DINNER: Mushroom and Spinach Stuffed Chicken Breast

DAY 9

BREAKFAST: Egg and Vegetable Breakfast Wrap

LUNCH: Mushroom and Spinach Quiche Cups

SNACK: Mango and Avocado Salsa

DINNER: Baked Lemon Garlic Chicken with Roasted Vegetables

DAY 10

BREAKFAST: Salmon and Avocado Breakfast Toast
LUNCH: Shrimp and Vegetable Stir-Fry
SNACK: Berry Spinach Protein Smoothie
DINNER: Coconut Lime Shrimp Stir-Fry

DAY 11

BREAKFAST: Mushroom and Spinach Omelet
LUNCH: Quinoa and Veggie Stuffed Bell Peppers
SNACK: Sweet Potato and Chickpea Patties
DINNER: Herb-Crusted Baked Salmon with Quinoa and Asparagus

DAY 12

BREAKFAST: Coconut-Berry Smoothie Bowl
LUNCH: Chicken and Avocado Wrap
SNACK: Cottage Cheese and Pineapple Stuffed Bell Peppers
DINNER: Mango Avocado Chicken Salad

DAY 13

BREAKFAST: Quinoa Breakfast Porridge

LUNCH: Eggplant and Lentil Curry

SNACK: Turmeric Roasted Chickpeas

DINNER: Turmeric Ginger Lentil Stew with Spinach

DAY 14

BREAKFAST: Cucumber and Smoked Salmon Roll-Ups

LUNCH: Caprese Avocado Salad

SNACK: Kale and Almond Butter Energy Balls

DINNER: Sesame Garlic Tofu Stir-Fry with Broccoli and Brown Rice

DAY 15

BREAKFAST: Pumpkin Spice Overnight Oats

LUNCH: Quinoa and Broccoli Buddha Bowl

SNACK: Avocado and Tomato Bruschetta

DINNER: Lemon Garlic Shrimp with Zucchini Noodles

DAY 16

BREAKFAST: Quinoa Breakfast Bowl

LUNCH: Quinoa Salad with Roasted Vegetables

SNACK: Hummus and Veggie Snack Platter

DINNER: Baked Chicken Breast with Sweet Potato and Asparagus

DAY 17

BREAKFAST: Avocado Toast with Poached Egg

LUNCH: Mediterranean Chickpea Bowl

SNACK: Apple Almond Energy Bites

DINNER: Lemon Garlic Shrimp Stir-Fry with Broccoli and Brown Rice

DAY 18

BREAKFAST: Greek Yogurt Parfait

LUNCH: Turkey and Quinoa Stuffed Bell Peppers

SNACK: Edamame and Avocado Salsa

DINNER: Vegetarian Lentil and Spinach Stuffed Bell Peppers

DAY 19

BREAKFAST: Oatmeal Banana Pancakes

LUNCH: Salmon and Vegetable Stir-Fry

SNACK: Roasted Chickpeas with Turmeric and Cumin

DINNER: Sesame Ginger Tofu Stir-Fry

DAY 20

BREAKFAST: Spinach and Feta Egg Muffins

LUNCH: Vegetarian Lentil and Vegetable Soup

SNACK: Spinach and Feta Stuffed Mushrooms

DINNER: Salmon and Quinoa Salad with Lemon Dill Dressing

DAY 21

BREAKFAST: Chia Seed Pudding with Berries

LUNCH: Quinoa and Chickpea Salad Bowl

SNACK: Almond Butter and Banana Rice Cakes

DINNER: Lemon Herb Baked Cod with Roasted Vegetables

DAY 22

BREAKFAST: Sweet Potato and Kale Breakfast Hash

LUNCH: Turkey and Vegetable Lettuce Wraps

SNACK: Cucumber Hummus Bites

DINNER: Vegetarian Lentil Curry with Quinoa

DAY 23

BREAKFAST: Cottage Cheese and Fruit Bowl

LUNCH: Sweet Potato and Black Bean Quinoa Bowl

SNACK: Zucchini and Walnut Muffins

DINNER: Mushroom and Spinach Stuffed Chicken Breast

DAY 24

BREAKFAST: Egg and Vegetable Breakfast Wrap

LUNCH: Mushroom and Spinach Quiche Cups

SNACK: Mango and Avocado Salsa

DINNER: Baked Lemon Garlic Chicken with Roasted Vegetables

DAY 25

BREAKFAST: Salmon and Avocado Breakfast Toast

LUNCH: Shrimp and Vegetable Stir-Fry

SNACK: Berry Spinach Protein Smoothie

DINNER: Coconut Lime Shrimp Stir-Fry

DAY 26

BREAKFAST: Mushroom and Spinach Omelet

LUNCH: Quinoa and Veggie Stuffed Bell Peppers

SNACK: Sweet Potato and Chickpea Patties

DINNER: Herb-Crusted Baked Salmon with Quinoa and Asparagus

DAY 27

BREAKFAST: Coconut-Berry Smoothie Bowl

LUNCH: Chicken and Avocado Wrap

SNACK: Cottage Cheese and Pineapple Stuffed Bell Peppers

DINNER: Mango Avocado Chicken Salad

DAY 28

BREAKFAST: Quinoa Breakfast Porridge
LUNCH: Eggplant and Lentil Curry
SNACK: Turmeric Roasted Chickpeas
DINNER: Turmeric Ginger Lentil Stew with Spinach

DAY 29

BREAKFAST: Cucumber and Smoked Salmon Roll-Ups
LUNCH: Caprese Avocado Salad
SNACK: Kale and Almond Butter Energy Balls
DINNER: Sesame Garlic Tofu Stir-Fry with Broccoli and Brown Rice

DAY 30

BREAKFAST: Pumpkin Spice Overnight Oats
LUNCH: Quinoa and Broccoli Buddha Bowl
SNACK: Avocado and Tomato Bruschetta
DINNER: Lemon Garlic Shrimp with Zucchini Noodles

CHAPTER 3: BREAKFASTS FOR ENERGY

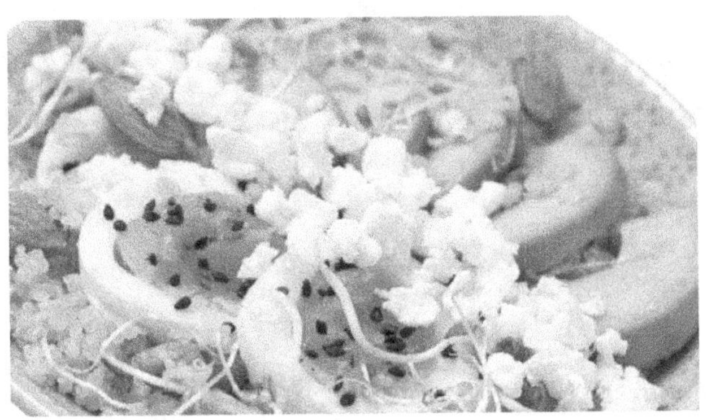

Quinoa Breakfast Bowl

Ingredients:

- 1 cup cooked quinoa
- 1/2 cup blueberries
- 1/2 cup sliced strawberries
- 1 tablespoon chia seeds
- 1 tablespoon honey
- 1/4 cup chopped almonds
- 1/2 cup almond milk (or any preferred milk)
- 1 teaspoon flaxseeds (optional)

Directions:

1. Cook quinoa according to package instructions.

2. In a bowl, combine cooked quinoa, blueberries, sliced strawberries, chia seeds, and chopped almonds.

3. Drizzle honey over the mixture and pour almond milk on top.

4. Mix well until all ingredients are evenly distributed.

5. Sprinkle flaxseeds on the top for an extra nutritional boost (optional).

6. Serve immediately and enjoy a nutritious, protein-packed breakfast.

Avocado Toast with Poached Egg

Ingredients:

- 1 slice whole-grain bread
- 1/2 ripe avocado
- 1 poached egg
- 1 teaspoon olive oil
- Salt and pepper to taste
- Optional toppings: cherry tomatoes, microgreens, or a sprinkle of turmeric.

Directions:

1. Toast the whole-grain bread to your liking.

2. While the bread is toasting, mash the ripe avocado in a bowl and add a pinch of salt and pepper.

3. Once the bread is toasted, spread the mashed avocado evenly on top.

4. Heat water in a pan until it's simmering. Crack an egg into a small bowl and gently slide it into the simmering water. Poach the egg for about 3-4 minutes.

5. Carefully remove the poached egg with a slotted spoon and place it on top of the avocado-covered toast.

6. Drizzle olive oil over the poached egg and avocado, and add any optional toppings you prefer.

7. Sprinkle with a bit more salt and pepper to taste.

Greek Yogurt Parfait

Ingredients:

- 1 cup Greek yogurt (unsweetened)
- 1/2 cup mixed berries (blueberries, raspberries, strawberries)
- 1 tablespoon honey or maple syrup
- 1/4 cup granola (choose a low-sugar, whole grain option)
- 1 tablespoon chopped nuts (almonds, walnuts, or your preference)
- 1/2 teaspoon chia seeds (optional)
- A sprinkle of cinnamon

Directions:

1. In a glass or bowl, start with a layer of Greek yogurt.

2. Add a layer of mixed berries on top of the yogurt.

3. Drizzle honey or maple syrup over the berries.

4. Sprinkle granola evenly on the berries layer.

5. Add another layer of Greek yogurt on top of the granola.

6. Sprinkle chopped nuts and chia seeds (if using) over the second yogurt layer.

7. Finish with another layer of mixed berries.

8. Sprinkle a bit of cinnamon over the top for extra flavor.

9. Serve immediately and enjoy this delicious and protein-packed parfait.

Oatmeal Banana Pancakes

Ingredients:

- 1 ripe banana, mashed
- 1/2 cup rolled oats
- 2 eggs
- 1/2 teaspoon baking powder
- 1/2 teaspoon vanilla extract
- Pinch of cinnamon
- 1 tablespoon coconut oil (for cooking)
- Fresh berries and a drizzle of honey for topping

Directions:

1. In a blender or food processor, combine the mashed banana, rolled oats, eggs, baking powder, vanilla extract, and cinnamon. Blend until you have a smooth batter.
2. Heat coconut oil in a non-stick skillet over medium heat.
3. Pour small amounts of the batter onto the skillet to form pancakes.
4. Cook for 2-3 minutes on each side or until golden brown.
5. Once cooked, stack the pancakes on a plate.
6. Top with fresh berries and drizzle with honey.
7. Serve warm and enjoy these nutritious oatmeal banana pancakes.

Spinach and Feta Egg Muffins

Ingredients:

- 4 large eggs
- 1 cup fresh spinach, chopped
- 1/4 cup feta cheese, crumbled
- 1/4 cup cherry tomatoes, diced
- 1/4 cup red bell pepper, diced
- Salt and pepper to taste
- Cooking spray or a bit of olive oil for greasing the muffin tin

Directions:

1. Preheat your oven to 350°F (175°C).
2. In a bowl, whisk the eggs and season with salt and pepper.
3. Add chopped spinach, feta cheese, diced tomatoes, and red bell pepper to the egg mixture. Mix well.
4. Grease a muffin tin with cooking spray or a small amount of olive oil.
5. Pour the egg and vegetable mixture evenly into the muffin cups.
6. Bake in the preheated oven for 15-20 minutes or until the egg muffins are set and slightly golden on top.
7. Allow them to cool for a few minutes before removing from the muffin tin.
8. Serve warm and enjoy these flavorful spinach and feta egg muffins.

Chia Seed Pudding with Berries

Ingredients:

- 3 tablespoons chia seeds
- 1 cup unsweetened almond milk (or any preferred milk)
- 1/2 teaspoon vanilla extract
- 1 tablespoon maple syrup or honey

- Mixed berries (strawberries, blueberries, raspberries) for topping
- Sliced almonds or coconut flakes for garnish (optional)

Directions:

1. In a bowl, combine chia seeds, almond milk, vanilla extract, and maple syrup. Stir well.
2. Let the mixture sit for 5 minutes, then stir again to prevent clumping.
3. Cover the bowl and refrigerate for at least 2 hours or overnight to allow the chia seeds to absorb the liquid and create a pudding-like consistency.
4. Once the chia pudding has set, give it a good stir.
5. Spoon the chia pudding into serving bowls or jars.
6. Top with mixed berries and garnish with sliced almonds or coconut flakes if desired.
7. Serve chilled and enjoy this nutrient-packed chia seed pudding for a refreshing breakfast.

Sweet Potato and Kale Breakfast Hash

Ingredients:

- 1 medium sweet potato, peeled and diced
- 1 cup kale, chopped
- 1/2 onion, finely chopped
- 2 eggs

- 1 tablespoon olive oil
- Salt and pepper to taste
- Optional: a sprinkle of paprika or cayenne for added flavor

Directions:

1. In a skillet, heat olive oil over medium heat.
2. Add finely chopped onions and sauté until translucent.
3. Add diced sweet potatoes to the skillet and cook until they are tender and slightly crispy on the edges.
4. Toss in chopped kale and continue to cook until the kale is wilted.
5. Create two wells in the sweet potato and kale mixture for the eggs.
6. Crack one egg into each well, cover the skillet, and let the eggs cook to your desired doneness.
7. Season with salt, pepper, and optional paprika or cayenne for added flavor.
8. Once the eggs are cooked, serve the breakfast hash hot.

Cottage Cheese and Fruit Bowl

Ingredients:

- 1 cup low-fat cottage cheese
- 1/2 cup fresh pineapple chunks
- 1/2 cup mango slices

- 1/4 cup pomegranate seeds
- 1 tablespoon chopped mint leaves
- 1 tablespoon flaxseeds or chia seeds (optional)
- Drizzle of honey or maple syrup (optional)

Directions:

1. In a bowl, spoon the low-fat cottage cheese as the base.
2. Add fresh pineapple chunks, mango slices, and pomegranate seeds on top.
3. Sprinkle chopped mint leaves over the fruit.
4. If desired, add flaxseeds or chia seeds for an extra nutritional boost.
5. Optionally, drizzle honey or maple syrup for sweetness.
6. Gently toss the ingredients together or enjoy in layers.
7. Serve chilled and savor this refreshing and protein-packed cottage cheese and fruit bowl.

Egg and Vegetable Breakfast Wrap

Ingredients:

- 2 large eggs, beaten
- 1 whole-grain or spinach tortilla
- 1/2 cup mixed vegetables (bell peppers, cherry tomatoes, spinach), diced
- 1 tablespoon feta cheese, crumbled
- 1 teaspoon olive oil

- Salt and pepper to taste

- Optional: salsa or avocado slices for serving

Directions:

1. Heat olive oil in a skillet over medium heat.

2. Add the mixed vegetables and sauté until they are tender-crisp.

3. Pour the beaten eggs over the vegetables in the skillet.

4. Gently scramble the eggs with the vegetables until fully cooked.

5. Sprinkle feta cheese over the egg and vegetable mixture, letting it melt slightly.

6. Season with salt and pepper to taste.

7. Warm the tortilla in the skillet or microwave for a few seconds.

8. Spoon the egg and vegetable mixture onto the center of the tortilla.

9. Optionally, add salsa or avocado slices for extra flavor.

10. Fold the sides of the tortilla and roll it into a wrap.

11. Serve immediately and enjoy this protein-packed and veggie-filled breakfast wrap.

Salmon and Avocado Breakfast Toast

Ingredients:

- 1 slice whole-grain bread or a gluten-free alternative

- 2 ounces smoked salmon

- 1/2 ripe avocado, mashed

- 1 teaspoon capers

- Fresh dill for garnish

- Lemon wedge for squeezing

- Salt and pepper to taste

Directions:

1. Toast the whole-grain bread to your liking.

2. Spread the mashed avocado evenly on the toasted bread.

3. Drape slices of smoked salmon over the mashed avocado.

4. Sprinkle capers over the salmon.

5. Season with salt and pepper to taste.

6. Garnish with fresh dill.

7. Squeeze a wedge of lemon over the top for added freshness.

8. Serve immediately and savor this nutrient-rich salmon and avocado breakfast toast.

Mushroom and Spinach Omelet

Ingredients:

- 2 large eggs

- 1/2 cup sliced mushrooms

- 1 cup fresh spinach, chopped

- 1/4 cup diced red bell pepper
- 1 tablespoon olive oil
- Salt and pepper to taste
- 2 tablespoons grated Parmesan cheese (optional)

Directions:

1. In a bowl, beat the eggs and season with salt and pepper.
2. Heat olive oil in a non-stick skillet over medium heat.
3. Add sliced mushrooms and diced red bell pepper to the skillet. Saute until they are tender.
4. Add chopped spinach to the skillet and cook until wilted.
5. Push the vegetables to one side of the skillet and pour the beaten eggs onto the other side.
6. Allow the eggs to set slightly, then gently stir them into the vegetables.
7. Cook until the eggs are fully set and the vegetables are evenly distributed.
8. If desired, sprinkle Parmesan cheese over one half of the omelette.
9. Fold the omelet in half and slide it onto a plate.
10. Serve hot and enjoy this protein-packed mushroom and spinach omelet.

Coconut-Berry Smoothie Bowl

Ingredients:

- 1 cup mixed berries (strawberries, blueberries, raspberries)
- 1 frozen banana, sliced
- 1/2 cup unsweetened coconut milk
- 1/4 cup Greek yogurt
- 2 tablespoons shredded coconut (unsweetened)
- 1 tablespoon chia seeds
- 1 tablespoon almond butter
- Optional toppings: additional berries, sliced almonds, or a drizzle of honey

Directions:

1. In a blender, combine mixed berries, frozen banana slices, coconut milk, Greek yogurt, shredded coconut, chia seeds, and almond butter.
2. Blend until smooth and creamy. Add more coconut milk if needed to reach your desired consistency.
3. Pour the smoothie into a bowl.
4. Top with additional berries, sliced almonds, or a drizzle of honey if desired.
5. Serve immediately and enjoy this refreshing and nutrient-packed coconut-berry smoothie bowl.

Quinoa Breakfast Porridge

Ingredients:

- 1/2 cup quinoa (rinsed)
- 1 cup almond milk (unsweetened)
- 1/2 teaspoon ground cinnamon
- 1/4 teaspoon vanilla extract
- 1 tablespoon chopped nuts (walnuts, almonds, or your choice)
- 1 tablespoon dried fruits (raisins, cranberries, or apricots)
- 1 tablespoon maple syrup or honey
- Fresh berries for topping

Directions:

1. In a saucepan, combine quinoa and almond milk. Bring to a gentle boil.
2. Reduce heat, add cinnamon, and simmer until quinoa is cooked and most of the liquid is absorbed (about 15 minutes).
3. Stir in vanilla extract, chopped nuts, and dried fruits.
4. Sweeten with maple syrup or honey, adjusting to your taste preference.
5. Remove from heat and let it sit for a minute to thicken.
6. Spoon the quinoa porridge into a bowl.
7. Top with fresh berries.

8. Serve warm and enjoy this protein-rich and fiber-filled quinoa breakfast porridge.

Cucumber and Smoked Salmon Roll-Ups

Ingredients:

- 1 medium cucumber
- 4 ounces smoked salmon
- 1/4 cup whipped cream cheese or Greek yogurt
- 1 tablespoon capers
- Fresh dill for garnish
- Lemon wedges for serving

Directions:

1. Using a vegetable peeler, thinly slice the cucumber lengthwise into long strips.
2. Lay out the cucumber slices on a clean surface.
3. Spread a thin layer of whipped cream cheese or Greek yogurt onto each cucumber slice.
4. Place a slice of smoked salmon on top of the cream cheese or yogurt.
5. Sprinkle capers evenly over the smoked salmon.
6. Carefully roll up each cucumber slice into a neat roll.
7. Secure with toothpicks if needed.
8. Garnish with fresh dill.

9. Serve with lemon wedges on the side for a touch of brightness.

10. Enjoy these refreshing and protein-packed cucumber and smoked salmon roll-ups.

Pumpkin Spice Overnight Oats

Ingredients:

- 1/2 cup rolled oats
- 1/2 cup canned pumpkin puree
- 1/2 cup unsweetened almond milk
- 1 tablespoon chia seeds
- 1/2 teaspoon pumpkin pie spice
- 1 tablespoon maple syrup or honey
- 1/4 cup chopped pecans or walnuts (optional)
- Greek yogurt for topping (optional)

Directions:

1. In a jar or container, combine rolled oats, pumpkin puree, almond milk, chia seeds, pumpkin pie spice, and maple syrup.

2. Stir well to ensure the ingredients are evenly mixed.

3. Cover the jar or container and refrigerate overnight or for at least 4 hours to allow the oats to absorb the liquid.

4. Before serving, give the mixture a good stir.

5. Top with chopped nuts and a dollop of Greek yogurt if desired.

6. Serve chilled and enjoy these flavorful pumpkin spice overnight oats.

Broccoli and Goat Cheese Frittata

Ingredients:

- 4 large eggs
- 1 cup broccoli florets, steamed or blanched
- 2 ounces goat cheese, crumbled
- 1/4 cup cherry tomatoes, halved
- 1/4 cup red onion, finely chopped
- 1 tablespoon olive oil
- Salt and pepper to taste
- Fresh basil or parsley for garnish

Directions:

1. Preheat your oven broiler.
2. In a bowl, whisk together the eggs and season with salt and pepper.
3. Heat olive oil in an oven-safe skillet over medium heat.
4. Add finely chopped red onion to the skillet and sauté until softened.

5. Add steamed or blanched broccoli florets and halved cherry tomatoes to the skillet. Cook for an additional 2-3 minutes.

6. Pour the whisked eggs over the vegetables in the skillet.

7. Allow the eggs to set around the edges, then sprinkle crumbled goat cheese evenly over the top.

8. Transfer the skillet to the preheated broiler and cook for 3-5 minutes or until the frittata is set and slightly golden on top.

9. Remove from the oven, garnish with fresh basil or parsley, and let it cool for a moment.

10. Slice and serve this delicious and protein-rich broccoli and goat cheese frittata.

Turkey and Vegetable Breakfast Burrito

Ingredients:

- 2 large eggs, scrambled
- 1 whole-grain or spinach tortilla
- 2 ounces lean turkey sausage or turkey bacon, cooked and crumbled
- 1/4 cup bell peppers (any color), diced
- 1/4 cup black beans, rinsed and drained
- 1 tablespoon salsa
- 1 tablespoon shredded cheddar cheese

- Fresh cilantro for garnish

Directions:

1. In a skillet, cook the lean turkey sausage or bacon until it's browned and cooked through. Remove from the skillet and crumble.

2. In the same skillet, add diced bell peppers and cook until they are slightly tender.

3. Add the scrambled eggs to the skillet and cook until just set.

4. Warm the tortilla in the skillet or microwave for a few seconds.

5. Assemble the burrito by placing the scrambled eggs, crumbled turkey sausage or bacon, black beans, salsa, and shredded cheddar cheese in the center of the tortilla.

6. Fold the sides of the tortilla and roll it into a burrito.

7. Garnish with fresh cilantro.

8. Serve immediately and enjoy this protein-packed and veggie-filled breakfast burrito.

Blueberry Almond Overnight Oats

Ingredients:

- 1/2 cup rolled oats
- 1/2 cup unsweetened almond milk
- 1/4 cup Greek yogurt

- 1/2 cup fresh blueberries
- 1 tablespoon almond butter
- 1 tablespoon chia seeds
- 1 teaspoon honey or maple syrup (optional)
- Sliced almonds for topping

Directions:

1. In a jar or container, combine rolled oats, almond milk, Greek yogurt, almond butter, chia seeds, and honey or maple syrup if desired.
2. Stir well to ensure all ingredients are evenly mixed.
3. Gently fold in fresh blueberries.
4. Cover the jar or container and refrigerate overnight or for at least 4 hours to allow the oats to absorb the liquid.
5. Before serving, give the mixture a good stir.
6. Top with sliced almonds.
7. Serve chilled and enjoy these flavorful blueberry almond overnight oats.

Chickpea and Spinach Breakfast Skillet

Ingredients:

- 1 can (15 oz) chickpeas, drained and rinsed
- 2 cups fresh spinach, chopped
- 1/2 cup cherry tomatoes, halved
- 1/4 cup red onion, finely chopped

- 2 cloves garlic, minced
- 2 tablespoons olive oil
- 1 teaspoon ground cumin
- Salt and pepper to taste
- 2 large eggs
- Fresh parsley for garnish

Directions:

1. In a skillet, heat olive oil over medium heat.
2. Add finely chopped red onion and minced garlic to the skillet. Sauté until softened.
3. Add chickpeas and cherry tomatoes to the skillet. Cook for 3-4 minutes.
4. Sprinkle ground cumin over the chickpea mixture and stir to coat evenly.
5. Add chopped spinach to the skillet and cook until wilted.
6. Create two wells in the mixture for the eggs.
7. Crack one egg into each well, cover the skillet, and let the eggs cook to your desired doneness.
8. Season with salt and pepper to taste.
9. Garnish with fresh parsley.
10. Serve hot, and enjoy this protein-rich and veggie-filled chickpea and spinach breakfast skillet.

Tomato and Basil Avocado Toast

Ingredients:

- 1 slice whole-grain bread or a gluten-free alternative
- 1/2 ripe avocado, mashed
- 1 medium tomato, sliced
- Fresh basil leaves
- 1 teaspoon olive oil
- Balsamic glaze for drizzling (optional)
- Salt and pepper to taste

Directions:

1. Toast the whole-grain bread to your liking.
2. Spread the mashed avocado evenly on the toasted bread.
3. Arrange tomato slices on top of the mashed avocado.
4. Tear fresh basil leaves and scatter them over the tomatoes.
5. Drizzle olive oil over the tomatoes and basil.
6. Optionally, add a few drops of balsamic glaze for extra flavor.
7. Sprinkle with salt and pepper to taste.
8. Serve immediately and enjoy this refreshing and nutrient-rich tomato and basil avocado toast.

CHAPTER 4: LUNCHES TO FUEL RECOVERY

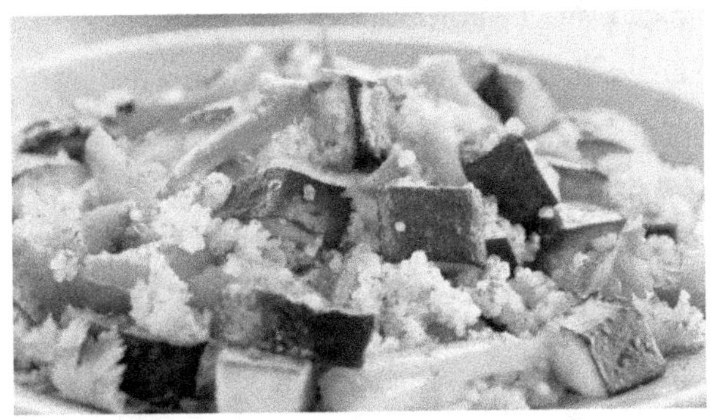

Quinoa Salad with Roasted Vegetables

Ingredients:

- 1 cup quinoa, rinsed
- 2 cups mixed vegetables (zucchini, cherry tomatoes, bell peppers)
- 1 tablespoon olive oil
- 1 teaspoon dried oregano
- 1/2 teaspoon garlic powder
- Salt and pepper to taste
- 1 can (15 oz) chickpeas, drained and rinsed
- 1/4 cup feta cheese, crumbled
- 2 tablespoons fresh lemon juice
- Fresh parsley for garnish

Directions:

1. Preheat the oven to 400°F (200°C).
2. In a bowl, toss the mixed vegetables with olive oil, dried oregano, garlic powder, salt, and pepper.
3. Spread the seasoned vegetables on a baking sheet in a single layer.
4. Roast in the preheated oven for 20-25 minutes or until the vegetables are tender and slightly caramelized.
5. While the vegetables are roasting, cook quinoa according to package instructions.
6. In a large bowl, combine cooked quinoa, roasted vegetables, chickpeas, and crumbled feta cheese.
7. Drizzle fresh lemon juice over the mixture and toss to combine.
8. Garnish with fresh parsley.
9. Season with additional salt and pepper if needed.
10. Serve the quinoa salad at room temperature or chilled.

Mediterranean Chickpea Bowl

Ingredients:

- 1 cup cooked quinoa or brown rice
- 1 can (15 oz) chickpeas, drained and rinsed
- 1 cup cherry tomatoes, halved
- 1 cucumber, diced

- 1/4 cup Kalamata olives, sliced
- 1/4 cup red onion, finely chopped
- 2 tablespoons feta cheese, crumbled
- 2 tablespoons extra-virgin olive oil
- 1 tablespoon balsamic vinegar
- Fresh parsley for garnish
- Salt and pepper to taste

Directions:

1. In a bowl, combine cooked quinoa or brown rice, chickpeas, cherry tomatoes, cucumber, Kalamata olives, red onion, and feta cheese.
2. In a small bowl, whisk together extra-virgin olive oil and balsamic vinegar to create the dressing.
3. Drizzle the dressing over the chickpea mixture and toss to coat evenly.
4. Season with salt and pepper to taste.
5. Garnish with fresh parsley.
6. Serve the Mediterranean chickpea bowl at room temperature or chilled.

Turkey and Quinoa Stuffed Bell Peppers

Ingredients:

- 4 bell peppers, halved and seeds removed
- 1 cup cooked quinoa

- 1/2 pound lean ground turkey
- 1 cup black beans, drained and rinsed
- 1 cup diced tomatoes
- 1/2 cup corn kernels
- 1/2 teaspoon cumin
- 1/2 teaspoon chili powder
- Salt and pepper to taste
- 1 cup shredded cheddar cheese
- Fresh cilantro for garnish

Directions:

1. Preheat the oven to 375°F (190°C).
2. In a skillet over medium heat, cook the ground turkey until browned. Season with cumin, chili powder, salt, and pepper.
3. In a large bowl, combine the cooked quinoa, black beans, diced tomatoes, corn, and the seasoned ground turkey.
4. Place the bell pepper halves in a baking dish.
5. Spoon the turkey and quinoa mixture into each bell pepper half.
6. Top each stuffed pepper with shredded cheddar cheese.
7. Cover the baking dish with foil and bake in the preheated oven for 25-30 minutes, or until the peppers are tender.

8. Remove the foil and bake for an additional 5 minutes or until the cheese is melted and bubbly.

9. Garnish with fresh cilantro.

10. Serve these turkey and quinoa stuffed bell peppers hot.

Salmon and Vegetable Stir-Fry

Ingredients:

- 2 salmon filets, skinless and boneless
- 2 cups broccoli florets
- 1 red bell pepper, sliced
- 1 carrot, julienned
- 2 tablespoons low-sodium soy sauce
- 1 tablespoon honey or maple syrup
- 1 tablespoon olive oil
- 2 cloves garlic, minced
- 1 teaspoon grated ginger
- Sesame seeds for garnish
- Green onions for garnish

Directions:

1. Cut the salmon into bite-sized pieces.

2. In a small bowl, whisk together soy sauce and honey or maple syrup to create the sauce.

3. Heat olive oil in a large skillet or wok over medium-high heat.

4. Add minced garlic and grated ginger to the skillet, sautéing for 30 seconds.

5. Add broccoli, red bell pepper, and julienned carrot to the skillet. Stir-fry for 3-4 minutes until the vegetables are slightly tender.

6. Push the vegetables to one side of the skillet and add the salmon pieces. Cook for 2-3 minutes per side until the salmon is cooked through.

7. Pour the sauce over the salmon and vegetables, tossing to coat evenly. Cook for an additional 1-2 minutes.

8. Garnish with sesame seeds and sliced green onions.

9. Serve the salmon and vegetable stir-fry hot over brown rice or quinoa.

Vegetarian Lentil and Vegetable Soup

Ingredients:

- 1 cup dried green or brown lentils, rinsed
- 1 onion, diced
- 2 carrots, sliced
- 2 celery stalks, chopped
- 2 cloves garlic, minced
- 1 can (14 oz) diced tomatoes
- 6 cups vegetable broth
- 1 teaspoon ground cumin

- 1/2 teaspoon smoked paprika
- Salt and pepper to taste
- 2 cups kale, chopped
- 1 tablespoon olive oil
- Fresh parsley for garnish
- Lemon wedges for serving

Directions:

1. In a large pot, heat olive oil over medium heat.

2. Add diced onion, sliced carrots, chopped celery, and minced garlic. Sauté until vegetables are softened.

3. Stir in dried lentils, diced tomatoes, vegetable broth, ground cumin, smoked paprika, salt, and pepper.

4. Bring the soup to a boil, then reduce the heat to low and let it simmer for about 25-30 minutes or until lentils are tender.

5. Add chopped kale to the soup and cook for an additional 5 minutes until the kale is wilted.

6. Adjust seasoning if needed.

7. Ladle the soup into bowls, garnish with fresh parsley.

8. Serve hot with lemon wedges on the side.

Quinoa and Chickpea Salad Bowl

Ingredients:

- 1 cup cooked quinoa

- 1 can (15 oz) chickpeas, drained and rinsed
- 1 cucumber, diced
- 1 cup cherry tomatoes, halved
- 1/4 cup red onion, finely chopped
- 1/4 cup feta cheese, crumbled
- 2 tablespoons extra-virgin olive oil
- 1 tablespoon balsamic vinegar
- 1 teaspoon Dijon mustard
- 1 teaspoon dried oregano
- Salt and pepper to taste
- Fresh parsley for garnish

Directions:

1. In a large bowl, combine cooked quinoa, chickpeas, diced cucumber, halved cherry tomatoes, chopped red onion, and crumbled feta cheese.
2. In a small bowl, whisk together extra-virgin olive oil, balsamic vinegar, Dijon mustard, dried oregano, salt, and pepper to create the dressing.
3. Drizzle the dressing over the salad mixture and toss to coat evenly.
4. Adjust seasoning if needed.
5. Garnish with fresh parsley.
6. Serve the quinoa and chickpea salad bowl at room temperature or chilled.

Turkey and Vegetable Lettuce Wraps

Ingredients:

- 1 pound lean ground turkey
- 1 tablespoon olive oil
- 1 onion, finely chopped
- 2 cloves garlic, minced
- 1 zucchini, diced
- 1 red bell pepper, diced
- 1 cup cherry tomatoes, quartered
- 1 teaspoon ground cumin
- 1 teaspoon smoked paprika
- Salt and pepper to taste
- Iceberg or butter lettuce leaves for wrapping
- 1/4 cup plain Greek yogurt (optional, for topping)
- Fresh cilantro for garnish

Directions:

1. In a large skillet, heat olive oil over medium heat.
2. Add finely chopped onion and minced garlic to the skillet. Sauté until softened.
3. Add ground turkey to the skillet and cook until browned.
4. Stir in diced zucchini, red bell pepper, and quartered cherry tomatoes.

5.   Season with ground cumin, smoked paprika, salt, and pepper. Cook for an additional 5-7 minutes until the vegetables are tender.
6.   Wash and separate the lettuce leaves to create wraps.
7.   Spoon the turkey and vegetable mixture into each lettuce leaf.
8.   Optionally, top with a dollop of plain Greek yogurt.
9.   Garnish with fresh cilantro.
10. Serve these turkey and vegetable lettuce wraps as a light and flavorful lunch.

Sweet Potato and Black Bean Quinoa Bowl

Ingredients:

- 1 cup quinoa, rinsed
- 2 medium sweet potatoes, peeled and diced
- 1 can (15 oz) black beans, drained and rinsed
- 1 cup corn kernels (fresh or frozen)
- 1 avocado, sliced
- 1/4 cup red onion, finely chopped
- 2 tablespoons cilantro, chopped
- 1 tablespoon olive oil
- 1 teaspoon ground cumin
- 1/2 teaspoon chili powder
- Salt and pepper to taste

- Lime wedges for serving

Directions:

1. Cook quinoa according to package instructions.

2. Preheat the oven to 400°F (200°C).

3. Toss diced sweet potatoes with olive oil, ground cumin, chili powder, salt, and pepper.

4. Spread the seasoned sweet potatoes on a baking sheet in a single layer.

5. Roast in the preheated oven for 20-25 minutes or until the sweet potatoes are tender and slightly caramelized.

6. In a bowl, combine cooked quinoa, black beans, corn, roasted sweet potatoes, chopped red onion, and cilantro.

7. Drizzle with additional olive oil and toss to combine.

8. Season with salt and pepper to taste.

9. Divide the mixture into bowls and top with sliced avocado.

10. Serve with lime wedges for a fresh burst of flavor.

Mushroom and Spinach Quiche Cups

Ingredients:

- 1 cup mushrooms, finely chopped
- 2 cups fresh spinach, chopped
- 1/2 cup cherry tomatoes, quartered
- 4 large eggs

- 1/2 cup milk (dairy or plant-based)
- 1/2 cup shredded cheese (cheddar, mozzarella, or your choice)
- 1 tablespoon olive oil
- 1/2 teaspoon dried thyme
- Salt and pepper to taste
- Cooking spray or olive oil for greasing muffin tin

Directions:

1. Preheat the oven to 375°F (190°C).
2. In a skillet, heat olive oil over medium heat.
3. Add chopped mushrooms and cook until they release their moisture and become golden brown.
4. Add chopped spinach to the skillet and cook until wilted.
5. In a bowl, whisk together eggs, milk, shredded cheese, dried thyme, salt, and pepper.
6. Grease a muffin tin with cooking spray or olive oil.
7. Divide the mushroom and spinach mixture among the muffin cups.
8. Pour the egg mixture over the vegetables in each muffin cup.
9. Top each quiche cup with quartered cherry tomatoes.
10. Bake in the preheated oven for 18-20 minutes or until the quiche cups are set and slightly golden.
11. Allow them to cool for a few minutes before serving.

Shrimp and Vegetable Stir-Fry

Ingredients:

- 1 pound shrimp, peeled and deveined
- 2 cups broccoli florets
- 1 red bell pepper, sliced
- 1 carrot, julienned
- 2 tablespoons low-sodium soy sauce
- 1 tablespoon honey or maple syrup
- 1 tablespoon olive oil
- 2 cloves garlic, minced
- 1 teaspoon grated ginger
- Sesame seeds for garnish
- Green onions for garnish
- Brown rice or quinoa for serving

Directions:

1. In a bowl, whisk together soy sauce and honey or maple syrup to create the sauce.

2. Heat olive oil in a large skillet or wok over medium-high heat.

3. Add minced garlic and grated ginger to the skillet, sautéing for 30 seconds.

4. Add shrimp to the skillet and cook for 2-3 minutes on each side until they turn pink and opaque. Remove from the skillet and set aside.

5. In the same skillet, add broccoli, red bell pepper, and julienned carrot. Stir-fry for 3-4 minutes until the vegetables are slightly tender.

6. Return the cooked shrimp to the skillet.

7. Pour the sauce over the shrimp and vegetables, tossing to coat evenly. Cook for an additional 1-2 minutes.

8. Garnish with sesame seeds and sliced green onions.

9. Serve the shrimp and vegetable stir-fry hot over brown rice or quinoa.

Quinoa and Veggie Stuffed Bell Peppers

Ingredients:

- 4 bell peppers, halved and seeds removed
- 1 cup quinoa, cooked according to package instructions
- 1 can (15 oz) black beans, drained and rinsed
- 1 cup corn kernels (fresh or frozen)
- 1 cup cherry tomatoes, diced
- 1/2 cup red onion, finely chopped
- 1 cup spinach, chopped
- 1 teaspoon ground cumin
- 1/2 teaspoon chili powder
- Salt and pepper to taste
- 1 cup shredded cheddar cheese
- Fresh cilantro for garnish

Directions:

1. Preheat the oven to 375°F (190°C).

2. In a large bowl, combine cooked quinoa, black beans, corn, diced cherry tomatoes, chopped red onion, chopped spinach, ground cumin, chili powder, salt, and pepper.

3. Mix well until all ingredients are evenly distributed.

4. Place the bell pepper halves in a baking dish.

5. Spoon the quinoa and vegetable mixture into each bell pepper half.

6. Top each stuffed pepper with shredded cheddar cheese.

7. Cover the baking dish with foil and bake in the preheated oven for 25-30 minutes or until the peppers are tender.

8. Remove the foil and bake for an additional 5 minutes or until the cheese is melted and bubbly.

9. Garnish with fresh cilantro.

10. Serve these quinoa and veggie stuffed bell peppers hot.

Chicken and Avocado Wrap

Ingredients:

- 2 boneless, skinless chicken breasts, cooked and sliced
- 1 avocado, sliced
- 1 cup cherry tomatoes, halved

- 1/4 cup red onion, finely chopped
- 1/4 cup Greek yogurt
- 1 tablespoon lime juice
- 1 teaspoon ground cumin
- Salt and pepper to taste
- Whole-grain wraps or tortillas
- Fresh cilantro for garnish

Directions:

1. In a bowl, mix Greek yogurt, lime juice, ground cumin, salt, and pepper to create the dressing.
2. Lay out the whole-grain wraps or tortillas.
3. Spread a generous spoonful of the dressing over each wrap.
4. Place slices of cooked chicken evenly on each wrap.
5. Add sliced avocado, halved cherry tomatoes, and chopped red onion.
6. Drizzle a little more dressing on top of the ingredients.
7. Garnish with fresh cilantro.
8. Fold the sides of the wraps and roll them tightly, securing the filling.
9. Slice in half if desired.
10. Serve these chicken and avocado wraps for a satisfying and easy-to-make lunch.

Eggplant and Lentil Curry

Ingredients:

- 1 large eggplant, diced
- 1 cup dry green or brown lentils, rinsed
- 1 can (14 oz) diced tomatoes
- 1 onion, finely chopped
- 2 cloves garlic, minced
- 1 tablespoon ginger, grated
- 1 can (14 oz) coconut milk
- 1 tablespoon curry powder
- 1 teaspoon ground cumin
- 1 teaspoon ground coriander
- 1/2 teaspoon turmeric
- Salt and pepper to taste
- 2 tablespoons olive oil
- Fresh cilantro for garnish
- Cooked brown rice or quinoa for serving

Directions:

1. In a large pot, heat olive oil over medium heat.
2. Add chopped onion, minced garlic, and grated ginger. Sauté until softened.
3. Add diced eggplant to the pot and cook for 5-7 minutes until it begins to soften.

4. Stir in curry powder, ground cumin, ground coriander, turmeric, salt, and pepper. Cook for an additional 2 minutes to toast the spices.

5. Add dry lentils, diced tomatoes, and coconut milk to the pot. Stir to combine.

6. Bring the mixture to a boil, then reduce the heat to low, cover, and simmer for 25-30 minutes or until lentils are tender.

7. Adjust seasoning if needed.

8. Serve the eggplant and lentil curry over cooked brown rice or quinoa.

9. Garnish with fresh cilantro.

Caprese Avocado Salad

Ingredients:

- 2 ripe avocados, diced
- 1 cup cherry tomatoes, halved
- 1 cup fresh mozzarella balls (or diced mozzarella)
- 1/4 cup fresh basil leaves, torn
- 2 tablespoons extra-virgin olive oil
- 1 tablespoon balsamic vinegar
- 1 teaspoon honey
- Salt and pepper to taste
- Whole-grain crackers or bread for serving (optional)

Directions:

1. In a large bowl, combine diced avocados, halved cherry tomatoes, fresh mozzarella balls, and torn basil leaves.

2. In a small bowl, whisk together extra-virgin olive oil, balsamic vinegar, honey, salt, and pepper to create the dressing.

3. Drizzle the dressing over the salad and gently toss to coat the ingredients evenly.

4. Adjust seasoning if needed.

5. Allow the salad to marinate for a few minutes to enhance flavors.

6. Serve the Caprese avocado salad on its own or with whole-grain crackers or bread.

Quinoa and Broccoli Buddha Bowl

Ingredients:

- 1 cup quinoa, rinsed
- 2 cups broccoli florets
- 1 cup edamame, shelled
- 1 carrot, julienned
- 1/4 cup tamari or low-sodium soy sauce
- 2 tablespoons sesame oil
- 1 tablespoon rice vinegar
- 1 tablespoon honey or maple syrup

- 1 teaspoon grated ginger
- 1 teaspoon sesame seeds
- Salt and pepper to taste
- Sliced avocado for garnish
- Chopped green onions for garnish

Directions:

1. Cook quinoa according to package instructions.

2. Steam broccoli florets until tender-crisp, about 4-5 minutes.

3. In a small bowl, whisk together tamari or soy sauce, sesame oil, rice vinegar, honey or maple syrup, grated ginger, sesame seeds, salt, and pepper to create the dressing.

4. In each bowl, assemble cooked quinoa, steamed broccoli, shelled edamame, and julienned carrot.

5. Drizzle the dressing over the bowl.

6. Garnish with sliced avocado and chopped green onions.

7. Toss gently to combine all the ingredients.

8. Serve this quinoa and broccoli Buddha bowl for a nutrient-packed and easy-to-make lunch.

Mango Chicken Salad Wrap

Ingredients:

- 1 cup cooked chicken breast, shredded or diced

- 1 mango, peeled, pitted, and diced
- 1/2 cup cucumber, diced
- 1/4 cup red bell pepper, finely chopped
- 2 tablespoons red onion, finely chopped
- 1/4 cup fresh cilantro, chopped
- 2 tablespoons Greek yogurt
- 1 tablespoon lime juice
- 1 teaspoon curry powder
- Salt and pepper to taste
- Whole-grain wraps or tortillas
- Fresh spinach leaves for filling

Directions:

1. In a bowl, combine shredded or diced cooked chicken, diced mango, diced cucumber, chopped red bell pepper, chopped red onion, and chopped cilantro.

2. In a small bowl, mix Greek yogurt, lime juice, curry powder, salt, and pepper to create the dressing.

3. Add the dressing to the chicken and mango mixture and toss until well combined.

4. Lay out the whole-grain wraps or tortillas.

5. Place fresh spinach leaves on each wrap.

6. Spoon the mango chicken salad onto the wraps.

7. Roll the wraps tightly, securing the filling.

8. Slice in half if desired.

9. Serve these mango chicken salad wraps for a delicious and easy-to-make lunch.

Spinach and Chickpea Quinoa Bowl

Ingredients:

- 1 cup quinoa, rinsed
- 2 cups fresh spinach leaves
- 1 can (15 oz) chickpeas, drained and rinsed
- 1 cup cherry tomatoes, halved
- 1/4 cup red onion, finely chopped
- 1/4 cup feta cheese, crumbled
- 2 tablespoons extra-virgin olive oil
- 1 tablespoon balsamic vinegar
- 1 teaspoon Dijon mustard
- 1 teaspoon dried oregano
- Salt and pepper to taste
- Sunflower seeds for garnish (optional)

Directions:

1. Cook quinoa according to package instructions.
2. In a large bowl, assemble fresh spinach leaves, cooked quinoa, chickpeas, halved cherry tomatoes, chopped red onion, and crumbled feta cheese.

3. In a small bowl, whisk together extra-virgin olive oil, balsamic vinegar, Dijon mustard, dried oregano, salt, and pepper to create the dressing.

4. Drizzle the dressing over the quinoa bowl and toss to coat evenly.

5. Adjust seasoning if needed.

6. Optionally, garnish with sunflower seeds for added crunch.

7. Serve the spinach and chickpea quinoa bowl as a nutrient-rich and easy-to-make lunch.

Salmon and Asparagus Quinoa Salad

Ingredients:

- 1 cup quinoa, rinsed
- 2 salmon filets
- 1 bunch asparagus, trimmed
- 1 tablespoon olive oil
- 1 lemon, zest and juice
- 2 cloves garlic, minced
- 1 teaspoon dried dill
- Salt and pepper to taste
- 1/4 cup cherry tomatoes, halved
- 1/4 cup cucumber, diced
- 1/4 cup red onion, finely chopped

- 2 tablespoons fresh parsley, chopped

Directions:

1. Cook quinoa according to package instructions.

2. Preheat the oven to 400°F (200°C).

3. Place salmon filets on a baking sheet lined with parchment paper. Drizzle with olive oil and sprinkle with minced garlic, dried dill, salt, and pepper. Add lemon zest on top.

4. Arrange trimmed asparagus around the salmon on the baking sheet. Drizzle with a bit of olive oil and season with salt and pepper.

5. Bake in the preheated oven for 12-15 minutes or until the salmon is cooked through and flakes easily with a fork.

6. In a large bowl, combine cooked quinoa, halved cherry tomatoes, diced cucumber, finely chopped red onion, and chopped fresh parsley.

7. Flake the baked salmon into bite-sized pieces and add it to the quinoa mixture.

8. Squeeze lemon juice over the salad and toss gently to combine.

9. Adjust seasoning if needed.

10. Serve the salmon and asparagus quinoa salad as a protein-rich and easy-to-make lunch.

Vegetarian Chickpea and Sweet Potato Bowl

Ingredients:

- 1 cup quinoa, rinsed
- 2 medium sweet potatoes, peeled and diced
- 1 can (15 oz) chickpeas, drained and rinsed
- 1 cup cherry tomatoes, halved
- 1 cup cucumber, diced
- 1/4 cup red onion, finely chopped
- 2 tablespoons olive oil
- 1 teaspoon ground cumin
- 1/2 teaspoon smoked paprika
- Salt and pepper to taste
- 1/4 cup tahini
- 2 tablespoons lemon juice
- 1 clove garlic, minced
- Fresh parsley for garnish

Directions:

1. Cook quinoa according to package instructions.
2. Preheat the oven to 400°F (200°C).
3. Toss diced sweet potatoes with olive oil, ground cumin, smoked paprika, salt, and pepper.
4. Spread the seasoned sweet potatoes on a baking sheet in a single layer.

5. Roast in the preheated oven for 20-25 minutes or until the sweet potatoes are tender and slightly caramelized.

6. In a bowl, combine cooked quinoa, roasted sweet potatoes, chickpeas, halved cherry tomatoes, diced cucumber, and finely chopped red onion.

7. In a small bowl, whisk together tahini, lemon juice, minced garlic, salt, and pepper to create the dressing.

8. Drizzle the tahini dressing over the bowl and toss to coat evenly.

9. Adjust seasoning if needed.

10. Garnish with fresh parsley.

11. Serve this vegetarian chickpea and sweet potato bowl for a nutrient-rich and easy-to-make lunch.

Teriyaki Salmon Rice Bowl

Ingredients:

- 2 salmon filets
- 1 cup brown rice, cooked
- 1 cup broccoli florets
- 1 carrot, julienned
- 1/4 cup low-sodium soy sauce
- 2 tablespoons honey or maple syrup
- 1 tablespoon rice vinegar
- 1 teaspoon grated ginger

- 1 clove garlic, minced

- 1 tablespoon sesame oil

- Sesame seeds for garnish

- Sliced green onions for garnish

Directions:

1. Preheat the oven to 400°F (200°C).

2. Place salmon filets on a baking sheet lined with parchment paper.

3. In a small bowl, whisk together low-sodium soy sauce, honey or maple syrup, rice vinegar, grated ginger, minced garlic, and sesame oil to create the teriyaki sauce.

4. Brush the teriyaki sauce over the salmon filets.

5. Roast in the preheated oven for 12-15 minutes or until the salmon is cooked through and flakes easily with a fork.

6. In the last 5 minutes of baking, add broccoli florets to the baking sheet to roast.

7. In a bowl, assemble cooked brown rice, teriyaki salmon, roasted broccoli, and julienned carrot.

8. Drizzle additional teriyaki sauce over the bowl.

9. Garnish with sesame seeds and sliced green onions.

10. Serve this teriyaki salmon rice bowl as a delicious and easy-to-make lunch.

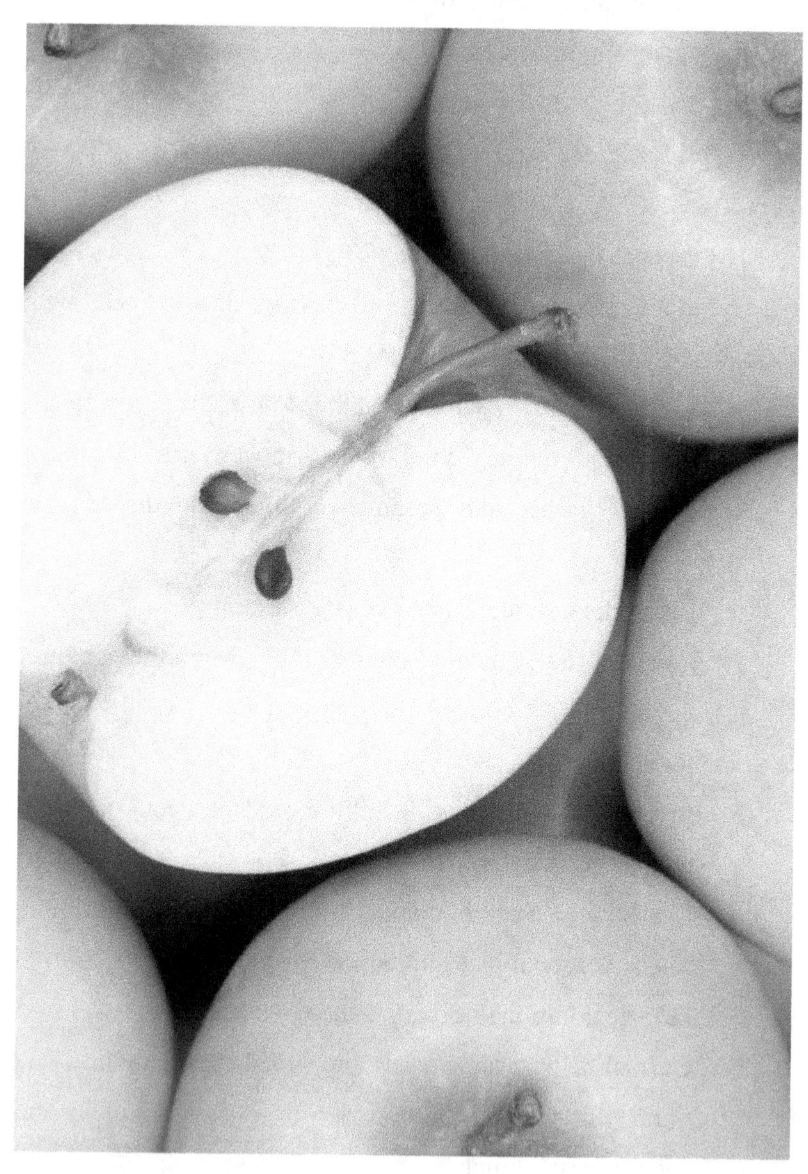

CHAPTER 5: HEALTHY SNACKS AND DESSERTS

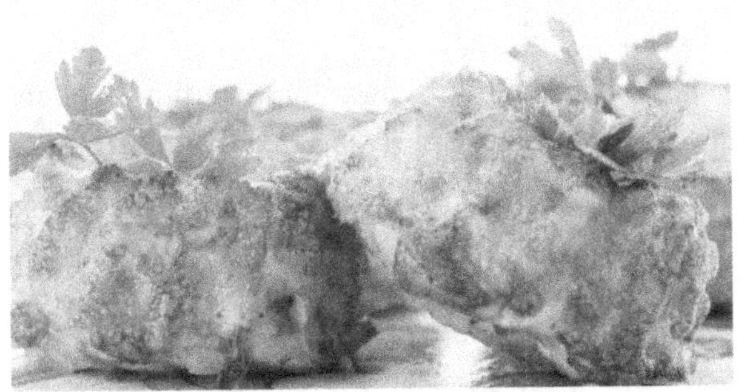

Hummus and Veggie Snack Platter

Ingredients:

- 1 cup hummus (store-bought or homemade)
- 1 cucumber, sliced
- 1 bell pepper (any color), sliced
- 2 medium carrots, peeled and sliced
- Cherry tomatoes
- Whole-grain pita bread or whole-grain crackers

Directions:

1. If you don't have store-bought hummus, you can make a simple homemade version by blending chickpeas, tahini, lemon juice, garlic, olive oil, and a pinch of salt in a food processor until smooth.

2. Arrange the hummus in the center of a serving platter.

3. Surround the hummus with cucumber slices, bell pepper slices, carrot slices, and cherry tomatoes.

4. Cut whole-grain pita bread into wedges or provide whole-grain crackers on the side.

5. Serve immediately and enjoy this delicious and nutritious hummus and veggie snack platter.

Apple Almond Energy Bites

Ingredients:

- 1 cup rolled oats
- 1/2 cup almond butter (unsweetened)
- 1/4 cup honey or maple syrup
- 1/2 cup finely chopped dried apples
- 1/4 cup chopped almonds
- 1 teaspoon cinnamon
- 1/2 teaspoon vanilla extract
- Pinch of salt

Directions:

1. In a mixing bowl, combine rolled oats, almond butter, honey or maple syrup, dried apples, chopped almonds, cinnamon, vanilla extract, and a pinch of salt.

2. Stir the mixture until all ingredients are well combined.

3. Place the bowl in the refrigerator for about 15-20 minutes to make the mixture easier to handle.

4. After chilling, take small portions of the mixture and roll them into bite-sized balls using your hands.

5. Place the energy bites on a parchment-lined tray or plate.

6. Refrigerate for at least 30 minutes to allow the bites to firm up.

7. Once firm, transfer the energy bites to an airtight container and store in the refrigerator.

8. Grab a couple of these Apple Almond Energy Bites for a quick and nutritious snack.

Edamame and Avocado Salsa

Ingredients:

- 1 cup cooked and shelled edamame
- 1 ripe avocado, diced
- 1/2 cup cherry tomatoes, quartered
- 1/4 cup red onion, finely chopped
- 1/4 cup fresh cilantro, chopped
- Juice of 1 lime
- 1 tablespoon olive oil
- Salt and pepper to taste
- Whole-grain tortilla chips or cucumber slices for serving

Directions:

1. In a bowl, combine cooked edamame, diced avocado, quartered cherry tomatoes, finely chopped red onion, and chopped cilantro.
2. In a small bowl, whisk together lime juice, olive oil, salt, and pepper to create the dressing.
3. Pour the dressing over the edamame and avocado mixture and gently toss to combine.
4. Adjust seasoning if needed.
5. Let the salsa sit for a few minutes to allow the flavors to meld.
6. Serve the Edamame and Avocado Salsa with whole-grain tortilla chips or cucumber slices for a refreshing and nutrient-rich snack.

Roasted Chickpeas with Turmeric and Cumin

Ingredients:

- 1 can (15 oz) chickpeas, drained and rinsed
- 1 tablespoon olive oil
- 1 teaspoon ground turmeric
- 1 teaspoon ground cumin
- 1/2 teaspoon smoked paprika
- 1/2 teaspoon garlic powder

- Salt and pepper to taste

Directions:

1. Preheat the oven to 400°F (200°C).
2. Pat the chickpeas dry with a paper towel to remove excess moisture.
3. In a bowl, toss chickpeas with olive oil, ground turmeric, ground cumin, smoked paprika, garlic powder, salt, and pepper until evenly coated.
4. Spread the seasoned chickpeas on a baking sheet in a single layer.
5. Roast in the preheated oven for 25-30 minutes or until the chickpeas are golden brown and crispy.
6. Shake the baking sheet halfway through the cooking time to ensure even roasting.
7. Remove from the oven and let the roasted chickpeas cool before serving.
8. Store in an airtight container for a crunchy and flavorful snack.

Spinach and Feta Stuffed Mushrooms

Ingredients:

- 12 large mushrooms, cleaned and stems removed
- 1 cup fresh spinach, chopped
- 1/2 cup feta cheese, crumbled

- 1/4 cup red bell pepper, finely chopped
- 1 clove garlic, minced
- 1 tablespoon olive oil
- Salt and pepper to taste
- Fresh parsley for garnish

Directions:

1. Preheat the oven to 375°F (190°C).
2. In a skillet, heat olive oil over medium heat. Add minced garlic and sauté for 1-2 minutes until fragrant.
3. Add chopped spinach and red bell pepper to the skillet. Cook until the spinach is wilted.
4. Remove the skillet from heat and let the mixture cool slightly.
5. In a bowl, combine the sautéed spinach and red bell pepper with crumbled feta cheese. Mix well.
6. Season the mixture with salt and pepper to taste.
7. Fill each mushroom cap with the spinach and feta mixture, pressing down gently.
8. Place the stuffed mushrooms on a baking sheet.
9. Bake in the preheated oven for 15-20 minutes or until the mushrooms are tender.
10. Garnish with fresh parsley before serving.

Almond Butter and Banana Rice Cakes

Ingredients:

- 4 brown rice cakes
- 1/2 cup almond butter (unsweetened)
- 2 ripe bananas, sliced
- 2 tablespoons chia seeds
- Drizzle of honey (optional)

Directions:

1. Spread almond butter evenly on each brown rice cake.
2. Top the almond butter with slices of ripe banana.
3. Sprinkle chia seeds over the banana slices.
4. Optional: Drizzle a bit of honey over the top for added sweetness.
5. Serve and enjoy these Almond Butter and Banana Rice Cakes as a quick and satisfying snack.

Cucumber Hummus Bites

Ingredients:

- 2 large cucumbers, sliced into rounds
- 1/2 cup hummus (store-bought or homemade)
- Cherry tomatoes, halved
- Kalamata olives, pitted and sliced
- Fresh dill or parsley for garnish

Directions:

1. Place cucumber rounds on a serving platter.

2. Spoon a small amount of hummus onto each cucumber round.

3. Top with halved cherry tomatoes and slices of Kalamata olives.

4. Garnish with fresh dill or parsley for added flavor.

5. Arrange the cucumber hummus bites on a platter and serve immediately.

Zucchini and Walnut Muffins

Ingredients:

- 1 1/2 cups grated zucchini (squeeze out excess moisture)
- 1 cup whole wheat flour
- 1/2 cup almond flour
- 1/4 cup coconut oil, melted
- 1/4 cup honey or maple syrup
- 2 eggs
- 1 teaspoon baking powder
- 1/2 teaspoon baking soda
- 1/2 teaspoon cinnamon
- 1/4 teaspoon salt
- 1/2 cup chopped walnuts
- Zest of 1 lemon

Directions:

1. Preheat the oven to 350°F (175°C) and line a muffin tin with paper liners.

2. In a large bowl, whisk together melted coconut oil, honey or maple syrup, and eggs.

3. Add grated zucchini to the wet ingredients and mix well.

4. In a separate bowl, combine whole wheat flour, almond flour, baking powder, baking soda, cinnamon, and salt.

5. Gradually add the dry ingredients to the wet ingredients, stirring until just combined.

6. Fold in chopped walnuts and lemon zest.

7. Spoon the batter into the prepared muffin tin, filling each cup about two-thirds full.

8. Bake for 18-22 minutes or until a toothpick inserted into the center comes out clean.

9. Allow the muffins to cool in the tin for a few minutes before transferring them to a wire rack to cool completely.

Mango and Avocado Salsa

Ingredients:

- 1 ripe mango, diced
- 1 avocado, diced
- 1/4 cup red onion, finely chopped

- 1/4 cup fresh cilantro, chopped
- Juice of 1 lime
- 1 small jalapeño, seeds removed and finely chopped (optional for spice)
- Salt and pepper to taste
- Whole-grain rice cakes or baked tortilla chips for serving

Directions:

1. In a bowl, combine diced mango, diced avocado, finely chopped red onion, chopped cilantro, lime juice, and optional jalapeño.
2. Gently toss the ingredients together until well mixed.
3. Season the salsa with salt and pepper to taste.
4. Allow the flavors to meld by refrigerating the salsa for about 15-20 minutes.
5. Serve the Mango and Avocado Salsa with whole-grain rice cakes or baked tortilla chips for a refreshing and nutrient-rich snack.

Berry Spinach Protein Smoothie

Ingredients:

- 1 cup fresh spinach leaves
- 1/2 cup mixed berries (such as blueberries, strawberries, and raspberries)
- 1/2 banana, frozen

- 1/2 cup Greek yogurt (unsweetened)

- 1/2 cup almond milk (unsweetened)

- 1 scoop vanilla protein powder (plant-based or whey, as per preference)

- Ice cubes (optional)

Directions:

1. Place fresh spinach, mixed berries, frozen banana, Greek yogurt, almond milk, and protein powder in a blender.

2. Blend until smooth and creamy.

3. If a thicker consistency is desired, add ice cubes and blend again until well incorporated.

4. Pour the smoothie into a glass and enjoy this nutrient-packed Berry Spinach Protein Smoothie.

Sweet Potato and Chickpea Patties

Ingredients:

- 1 cup cooked sweet potato, mashed

- 1 can (15 oz) chickpeas, drained and rinsed

- 1/4 cup red onion, finely chopped

- 2 cloves garlic, minced

- 2 tablespoons fresh cilantro, chopped

- 1 teaspoon ground cumin

- 1/2 teaspoon smoked paprika

- Salt and pepper to taste

- 2 tablespoons olive oil (for cooking)
- Greek yogurt or tzatziki sauce for dipping

Directions:

1. In a large bowl, mash the cooked sweet potato and add chickpeas. Mash the chickpeas until a chunky mixture forms.
2. Add red onion, minced garlic, chopped cilantro, ground cumin, smoked paprika, salt, and pepper to the bowl. Mix well.
3. Form the mixture into small patties, about 2 inches in diameter.
4. Heat olive oil in a skillet over medium heat.
5. Cook the patties for 3-4 minutes on each side or until golden brown and cooked through.
6. Once cooked, transfer the patties to a plate lined with paper towels to absorb any excess oil.
7. Serve the Sweet Potato and Chickpea Patties with a side of Greek yogurt or tzatziki sauce for dipping.

Cottage Cheese and Pineapple Stuffed Bell Peppers

Ingredients:

- 2 large bell peppers, halved and seeds removed
- 1 cup low-fat cottage cheese

- 1/2 cup pineapple chunks, finely chopped
- 2 tablespoons fresh mint, chopped
- 1 tablespoon honey
- 1/4 cup chopped almonds (optional for crunch)
- Pinch of black pepper

Directions:

1. In a bowl, combine low-fat cottage cheese, finely chopped pineapple, fresh mint, and honey. Mix well.
2. If desired, add chopped almonds for an extra crunch and fold them into the mixture.
3. Season the filling with a pinch of black pepper to taste.
4. Spoon the cottage cheese and pineapple mixture into each halved bell pepper.
5. Chill in the refrigerator for about 15-20 minutes to let the flavors meld.
6. Serve these Cottage Cheese and Pineapple Stuffed Bell Peppers as a refreshing and protein-rich snack.

Turmeric Roasted Chickpeas

Ingredients:

- 1 can (15 oz) chickpeas, drained and rinsed
- 1 tablespoon olive oil
- 1 teaspoon ground turmeric
- 1/2 teaspoon ground cumin

- 1/2 teaspoon smoked paprika
- 1/4 teaspoon cayenne pepper (adjust to taste)
- Salt to taste

Directions:

1. Preheat the oven to 400°F (200°C) and line a baking sheet with parchment paper.
2. In a bowl, toss the drained and rinsed chickpeas with olive oil until evenly coated.
3. In a separate small bowl, mix together ground turmeric, ground cumin, smoked paprika, cayenne pepper, and salt.
4. Sprinkle the spice mixture over the chickpeas, tossing to ensure they are well coated.
5. Spread the chickpeas in a single layer on the prepared baking sheet.
6. Roast in the preheated oven for 25-30 minutes or until golden brown and crispy, shaking the pan halfway through for even roasting.
7. Remove from the oven and let the roasted chickpeas cool before serving.

Kale and Almond Butter Energy Balls

Ingredients:

- 1 cup kale leaves, stems removed

- 1 cup pitted dates

- 1/2 cup almond butter (unsweetened)

- 1/4 cup unsweetened shredded coconut

- 1/4 cup raw almonds

- 1 tablespoon chia seeds

- 1/2 teaspoon vanilla extract

- Pinch of sea salt

Directions:

1. In a food processor, pulse kale until finely chopped.

2. Add pitted dates, almond butter, shredded coconut, raw almonds, chia seeds, vanilla extract, and a pinch of sea salt to the food processor.

3. Blend the ingredients until a sticky dough forms.

4. Scoop out small portions of the mixture and roll into bite-sized energy balls.

5. Place the energy balls on a parchment-lined tray.

6. Refrigerate for at least 30 minutes to allow the balls to firm up.

7. Once chilled, transfer the Kale and Almond Butter Energy Balls to an airtight container and store in the refrigerator.

Avocado and Tomato Bruschetta

Ingredients:

- 2 ripe avocados, diced
- 1 cup cherry tomatoes, diced
- 1/4 cup red onion, finely chopped
- 2 tablespoons fresh basil, chopped
- 1 clove garlic, minced
- 1 tablespoon balsamic vinegar
- 1 tablespoon olive oil
- Salt and pepper to taste
- Whole-grain baguette slices or whole-grain crackers for serving

Directions:

1. In a bowl, combine diced avocados, diced cherry tomatoes, finely chopped red onion, chopped fresh basil, and minced garlic.
2. Drizzle balsamic vinegar and olive oil over the mixture.
3. Gently toss the ingredients until well combined.
4. Season with salt and pepper to taste.
5. Let the Avocado and Tomato Bruschetta sit for a few minutes to allow the flavors to meld.
6. Serve the bruschetta on whole-grain baguette slices or alongside whole-grain crackers for a flavorful and nutrient-rich snack.

Banana-Oat Cookies

Ingredients:

- 2 ripe bananas, mashed
- 1 cup old-fashioned oats
- 1/4 cup almond butter (unsweetened)
- 1/4 cup chopped nuts (such as walnuts or almonds)
- 1/4 cup raisins or dried cranberries
- 1/2 teaspoon ground cinnamon
- 1/2 teaspoon vanilla extract
- Pinch of salt

Directions:

1. Preheat the oven to 350°F (175°C) and line a baking sheet with parchment paper.
2. In a bowl, combine mashed bananas, old-fashioned oats, almond butter, chopped nuts, raisins or dried cranberries, ground cinnamon, vanilla extract, and a pinch of salt.
3. Mix well until all ingredients are thoroughly combined.
4. Drop spoonfuls of the mixture onto the prepared baking sheet, shaping them into cookies.
5. Bake in the preheated oven for 12-15 minutes or until the edges turn golden brown.
6. Allow the cookies to cool on the baking sheet for a few minutes before transferring them to a wire rack to cool completely.

7. Once cooled, store the Banana-Oat Cookies in an airtight container.

Mango Coconut Rice Pudding

Ingredients:

- 1 cup cooked brown rice
- 1 ripe mango, diced
- 1 can (14 oz) coconut milk (unsweetened)
- 2 tablespoons honey or maple syrup
- 1/2 teaspoon vanilla extract
- 1/4 teaspoon ground cardamom
- Unsweetened shredded coconut for garnish (optional)

Directions:

1. In a saucepan, combine cooked brown rice, diced mango, coconut milk, honey or maple syrup, vanilla extract, and ground cardamom.
2. Stir well and bring the mixture to a gentle simmer over medium heat.
3. Reduce the heat to low and let it simmer for 15-20 minutes, stirring occasionally, until the pudding thickens.
4. Remove from heat and let it cool for a few minutes.
5. Optionally, garnish with unsweetened shredded coconut before serving.

6. Serve the Mango Coconut Rice Pudding warm or chilled.

Baked Peaches with Honey and Almonds

Ingredients:

- 4 ripe peaches, halved and pitted
- 2 tablespoons honey
- 1/4 cup sliced almonds
- 1/2 teaspoon ground cinnamon
- Greek yogurt or low-fat vanilla ice cream for serving (optional)

Directions:

1. Preheat the oven to 375°F (190°C) and line a baking dish with parchment paper.
2. Place the peach halves, cut side up, in the baking dish.
3. Drizzle honey over each peach half.
4. Sprinkle sliced almonds evenly over the peaches.
5. Dust the tops with ground cinnamon.
6. Bake in the preheated oven for 20-25 minutes or until the peaches are tender and the almonds are golden.
7. Remove from the oven and let them cool for a few minutes.
8. Optionally, serve the Baked Peaches with a dollop of Greek yogurt or a scoop of low-fat vanilla ice cream.

Frozen Banana Bites

Ingredients:

- 2 ripe bananas
- 1/4 cup natural almond butter (unsweetened)
- 1/4 cup dark chocolate chips (70% cocoa or higher)
- 1 tablespoon coconut oil
- Chopped nuts or shredded coconut for coating (optional)

Directions:

1. Peel and slice the bananas into bite-sized rounds.
2. Spread a small amount of almond butter on half of the banana slices and top with the remaining slices to create banana sandwiches.
3. Place the banana sandwiches on a parchment-lined tray and freeze for at least 1 hour.
4. In a microwave-safe bowl, melt the dark chocolate chips and coconut oil in 30-second intervals, stirring until smooth.
5. Dip each frozen banana bite into the melted chocolate, ensuring it's evenly coated.
6. Optionally, roll the chocolate-coated banana bites in chopped nuts or shredded coconut for added texture.
7. Place the coated banana bites back on the parchment-lined tray and return to the freezer for an additional 30 minutes or until the chocolate is set.

8. Once fully set, transfer the Frozen Banana Bites to an airtight container and store in the freezer.

Quinoa Pudding with Mixed Berries

Ingredients:

- 1/2 cup quinoa, rinsed
- 1 cup almond milk (unsweetened)
- 2 tablespoons honey or maple syrup
- 1/2 teaspoon vanilla extract
- 1/2 teaspoon ground cinnamon
- 1 cup mixed berries (blueberries, strawberries, raspberries)
- Chopped nuts for garnish (optional)

Directions:

1. In a saucepan, combine quinoa and almond milk. Bring to a boil, then reduce heat to low, cover, and simmer for 15-20 minutes or until quinoa is cooked and the mixture thickens.
2. Stir in honey or maple syrup, vanilla extract, and ground cinnamon.
3. Allow the quinoa pudding to cool for a few minutes.
4. In serving bowls, layer the quinoa pudding with mixed berries.
5. Optionally, garnish with chopped nuts for added texture.

6. Serve the Quinoa Pudding with Mixed Berries warm or chilled.

Apple Cinnamon Oat Bars

Ingredients:

- 2 cups rolled oats
- 1 cup unsweetened applesauce
- 1/4 cup almond butter (unsweetened)
- 1/4 cup honey or maple syrup
- 1 teaspoon ground cinnamon
- 1/2 teaspoon vanilla extract
- 1/2 cup diced apples (peeled)
- 1/4 cup chopped walnuts or almonds (optional)

Directions:

1. Preheat the oven to 350°F (175°C) and line a baking dish with parchment paper.
2. In a large bowl, combine rolled oats, applesauce, almond butter, honey or maple syrup, ground cinnamon, and vanilla extract. Mix until well combined.
3. Fold in diced apples and chopped nuts if using.
4. Press the mixture evenly into the prepared baking dish.
5. Bake in the preheated oven for 20-25 minutes or until the edges turn golden brown.

6. Allow the bars to cool in the dish before cutting them into squares or rectangles.

7. Once cooled, store the Apple Cinnamon Oat Bars in an airtight container.

Coconut Berry Parfait

Ingredients:

- 1 cup mixed berries (strawberries, blueberries, raspberries)
- 1 cup coconut yogurt (unsweetened)
- 2 tablespoons shredded coconut (unsweetened)
- 1 tablespoon chia seeds
- 1 tablespoon honey or maple syrup (optional, depending on sweetness preference)
- Fresh mint leaves for garnish (optional)

Directions:

1. In a bowl, combine coconut yogurt, shredded coconut, chia seeds, and honey or maple syrup if using. Mix well.

2. In serving glasses or bowls, layer the coconut yogurt mixture with mixed berries.

3. Repeat the layers until the glasses are filled, finishing with a layer of berries on top.

4. Optionally, garnish with fresh mint leaves.

5. Refrigerate for at least 30 minutes to allow the flavors to meld.

6. Serve the Coconut Berry Parfait chilled.

Pumpkin Spice Chia Pudding

Ingredients:

- 1/4 cup chia seeds
- 1 cup almond milk (unsweetened)
- 1/2 cup canned pumpkin puree
- 2 tablespoons maple syrup
- 1/2 teaspoon pumpkin spice blend
- 1/2 teaspoon vanilla extract
- Chopped pecans or walnuts for garnish (optional)

Directions:

1. In a bowl, whisk together chia seeds, almond milk, pumpkin puree, maple syrup, pumpkin spice blend, and vanilla extract.

2. Continue whisking for a few minutes to prevent clumping.

3. Cover the bowl and refrigerate for at least 2 hours or overnight until the chia pudding thickens.

4. Before serving, give the pudding a good stir.

5. Spoon the Pumpkin Spice Chia Pudding into serving glasses.

6. Optionally, garnish with chopped pecans or walnuts for added texture.

7. Serve and enjoy this seasonal and nutritious dessert.

CHAPTER 6: NOURISHING DINNERS

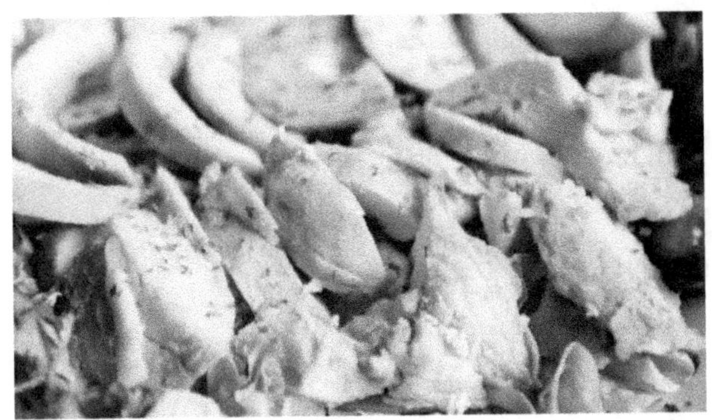

Baked Chicken Breast with Sweet Potato and Asparagus

Ingredients:

For Baked Chicken:

- 4 boneless, skinless chicken breasts
- 2 tablespoons olive oil
- 1 teaspoon paprika
- 1 teaspoon garlic powder
- Salt and pepper to taste

For Sweet Potato Mash:

- 2 large sweet potatoes, peeled and diced
- 2 tablespoons Greek yogurt (unsweetened)
- 1 tablespoon olive oil
- Salt and pepper to taste

For Asparagus:

- 1 bunch asparagus, trimmed
- 1 tablespoon balsamic vinegar
- 1 tablespoon olive oil
- Salt and pepper to taste

Directions:

Baked Chicken:

1. Preheat the oven to 400°F (200°C).
2. Place chicken breasts on a baking sheet.
3. In a small bowl, mix olive oil, paprika, garlic powder, salt, and pepper.
4. Brush the chicken breasts with the spice mixture.
5. Bake in the preheated oven for 20-25 minutes or until the internal temperature reaches 165°F (74°C).

Sweet Potato Mash:

1. Boil diced sweet potatoes until tender.
2. Drain and mash the sweet potatoes.
3. Stir in Greek yogurt, olive oil, salt, and pepper. Mix until smooth.

Asparagus:

1. Preheat the oven to 400°F (200°C).
2. Toss trimmed asparagus with balsamic vinegar, olive oil, salt, and pepper.

3. Spread the asparagus on a baking sheet and roast for 10-12 minutes or until tender-crisp.

Assembly:

1. Serve the baked chicken breast over a dollop of sweet potato mash.

2. Arrange the roasted asparagus on the side.

Lemon Garlic Shrimp Stir-Fry with Broccoli and Brown Rice

Ingredients:

For Shrimp:

- 1 pound large shrimp, peeled and deveined
- 2 tablespoons olive oil
- 3 cloves garlic, minced
- Zest and juice of 1 lemon
- 1 teaspoon dried oregano
- Salt and pepper to taste

For Stir-Fry:

- 4 cups broccoli florets
- 1 red bell pepper, thinly sliced
- 1 tablespoon low-sodium soy sauce
- 1 tablespoon sesame oil
- 2 cups cooked brown rice

Directions:

Shrimp:

1. In a bowl, mix shrimp with olive oil, minced garlic, lemon zest, lemon juice, dried oregano, salt, and pepper. Allow it to marinate for 15-20 minutes.

2. Heat a large skillet over medium-high heat. Add the marinated shrimp and cook for 2-3 minutes on each side until they turn pink and opaque. Remove the shrimp from the skillet and set aside.

Stir-Fry:

1. In the same skillet, add a bit more olive oil if needed. Stir in broccoli florets and red bell pepper slices.

2. Cook the vegetables for 5-7 minutes until they are tender-crisp.

3. Add the cooked shrimp back to the skillet.

4. Drizzle soy sauce and sesame oil over the shrimp and vegetables. Toss everything together until well coated.

Assembly:

1. Serve the lemon garlic shrimp stir-fry over a bed of cooked brown rice.

Vegetarian Lentil and Spinach Stuffed Bell Peppers

Ingredients:

- 4 bell peppers (any color)
- 1 cup dry green or brown lentils, rinsed
- 2.5 cups vegetable broth or water
- 1 tablespoon olive oil
- 1 onion, finely chopped
- 2 cloves garlic, minced
- 1 can (14 oz) diced tomatoes, drained
- 2 cups fresh spinach, chopped
- 1 teaspoon ground cumin
- 1 teaspoon smoked paprika
- Salt and pepper to taste
- 1 cup shredded mozzarella or your favorite cheese

Directions:

1. Preheat the oven to 375°F (190°C).
2. Cut the tops off the bell peppers and remove the seeds and membranes.
3. In a saucepan, combine lentils and vegetable broth or water. Bring to a boil, then reduce heat to low, cover, and simmer for 20-25 minutes or until lentils are tender.
4. In a large skillet, heat olive oil over medium heat. Add chopped onion and garlic, sauté until softened.

5. Stir in cooked lentils, drained diced tomatoes, chopped spinach, ground cumin, smoked paprika, salt, and pepper. Cook for an additional 5 minutes.

6. Fill each bell pepper with the lentil and spinach mixture.

7. Sprinkle shredded cheese on top of each stuffed pepper.

8. Place the stuffed peppers in a baking dish and bake in the preheated oven for 25-30 minutes or until the peppers are tender and the cheese is melted and bubbly.

9. Remove from the oven and let them cool for a few minutes before serving.

Sesame Ginger Tofu Stir-Fry

Ingredients:

For Tofu:

- 1 block extra-firm tofu, pressed and cubed
- 2 tablespoons soy sauce (low sodium)
- 1 tablespoon sesame oil
- 1 tablespoon rice vinegar
- 1 teaspoon grated ginger
- 1 teaspoon minced garlic
- 1 tablespoon cornstarch

For Stir-Fry:

- 2 tablespoons vegetable oil
- 1 cup broccoli florets

- 1 red bell pepper, thinly sliced
- 1 carrot, julienned
- 1 cup snap peas, ends trimmed
- 2 green onions, sliced
- 2 tablespoons soy sauce (low sodium)
- 1 tablespoon hoisin sauce
- 1 tablespoon sesame seeds (for garnish)
- Cooked brown rice or quinoa for serving

Directions:

Tofu:

1. In a bowl, whisk together soy sauce, sesame oil, rice vinegar, grated ginger, minced garlic, and cornstarch.
2. Add cubed tofu to the marinade, ensuring the tofu is well coated. Let it marinate for 15-20 minutes.

Stir-Fry:

1. Heat vegetable oil in a large skillet or wok over medium-high heat.
2. Add marinated tofu cubes and cook until golden brown on all sides. Remove from the skillet and set aside.
3. In the same skillet, add a bit more oil if needed. Stir in broccoli, red bell pepper, julienned carrot, and snap peas.
4. Cook the vegetables for 5-7 minutes until they are tender-crisp.
5. Add cooked tofu back to the skillet.

6. In a small bowl, mix soy sauce and hoisin sauce. Pour the sauce over the tofu and vegetables. Toss everything together until well coated.

7. Cook for an additional 2-3 minutes until heated through.

8. Serve the Sesame Ginger Tofu Stir-Fry over cooked brown rice or quinoa.

9. Garnish with sliced green onions and sesame seeds.

Salmon and Quinoa Salad with Lemon Dill Dressing

Ingredients:

For Salmon:

- 4 salmon filets (wild-caught)
- 2 tablespoons olive oil
- 1 teaspoon dried dill
- 1 teaspoon garlic powder
- Salt and pepper to taste
- Juice of 1 lemon

For Quinoa Salad:

- 1 cup quinoa, rinsed
- 2 cups vegetable broth or water
- 1 cucumber, diced
- 1 cup cherry tomatoes, halved
- 1/4 cup red onion, finely chopped

- 1/4 cup feta cheese, crumbled

- 2 tablespoons fresh dill, chopped

For Lemon Dill Dressing:

- 3 tablespoons olive oil

- Juice of 1 lemon

- 1 tablespoon Dijon mustard

- 1 teaspoon honey or maple syrup

- Salt and pepper to taste

Directions:

Salmon:

1. Preheat the oven to 400°F (200°C).

2. Place salmon filets on a baking sheet.

3. In a bowl, mix olive oil, dried dill, garlic powder, salt, and pepper. Brush the mixture over the salmon fillets.

4. Squeeze lemon juice over the salmon.

5. Bake in the preheated oven for 12-15 minutes or until the salmon is cooked through and flakes easily with a fork.

Quinoa Salad:

1. In a saucepan, combine quinoa and vegetable broth or water. Bring to a boil, then reduce heat to low, cover, and simmer for 15-20 minutes or until quinoa is cooked and the liquid is absorbed.

2. Fluff the quinoa with a fork and let it cool.

3. In a large bowl, combine cooled quinoa, diced cucumber, halved cherry tomatoes, chopped red onion, feta cheese, and fresh dill.

Lemon Dill Dressing:

1. In a small bowl, whisk together olive oil, lemon juice, Dijon mustard, honey or maple syrup, salt, and pepper.

Assembly:

1. Place the quinoa salad on a serving platter.
2. Top with baked salmon fillets.
3. Drizzle the Lemon Dill Dressing over the salmon and salad.
4. Serve and enjoy this refreshing and protein-packed dinner.

Lemon Herb Baked Cod with Roasted Vegetables

Ingredients:

For Baked Cod:

- 4 cod filets
- 2 tablespoons olive oil
- Zest and juice of 1 lemon
- 2 cloves garlic, minced
- 1 teaspoon dried thyme
- 1 teaspoon dried rosemary

- Salt and pepper to taste

For Roasted Vegetables:

- 2 cups baby potatoes, halved
- 2 cups baby carrots
- 1 cup cherry tomatoes, halved
- 1 tablespoon olive oil
- Salt and pepper to taste
- Fresh parsley for garnish

Directions:

Baked Cod:

1. Preheat the oven to 400°F (200°C).
2. Place cod filets on a baking sheet.
3. In a small bowl, mix olive oil, lemon zest, lemon juice, minced garlic, dried thyme, dried rosemary, salt, and pepper.
4. Brush the cod filets with the herb-infused mixture.
5. Bake in the preheated oven for 12-15 minutes or until the cod is opaque and flakes easily.

Roasted Vegetables:

1. In a separate baking dish, toss halved baby potatoes, baby carrots, and cherry tomatoes with olive oil, salt, and pepper.
2. Roast the vegetables in the oven for 20-25 minutes or until they are tender.

Assembly:

1. Arrange the baked cod filets on a serving plate.
2. Surround the cod with the roasted vegetables.
3. Garnish with fresh parsley for added flavor.

Vegetarian Lentil Curry with Quinoa

Ingredients:

- 1 cup dry green or brown lentils, rinsed
- 2 cups vegetable broth or water
- 1 tablespoon olive oil
- 1 onion, finely chopped
- 3 cloves garlic, minced
- 1 tablespoon ginger, grated
- 2 tablespoons curry powder
- 1 teaspoon ground cumin
- 1 teaspoon ground coriander
- 1 can (14 oz) diced tomatoes, undrained
- 1 can (14 oz) coconut milk
- Salt and pepper to taste
- Fresh cilantro for garnish
- Cooked quinoa for serving

Directions:

1. In a saucepan, combine lentils and vegetable broth or water. Bring to a boil, then reduce heat to low, cover, and simmer for 20-25 minutes or until lentils are tender.

2. In a large skillet, heat olive oil over medium heat. Add chopped onion and sauté until softened.

3. Add minced garlic and grated ginger to the skillet. Sauté for an additional 1-2 minutes until fragrant.

4. Stir in curry powder, ground cumin, and ground coriander. Cook for another 1-2 minutes.

5. Add diced tomatoes (with their juice) to the skillet. Simmer for 5 minutes.

6. Pour in the coconut milk and cooked lentils. Season with salt and pepper. Simmer for an additional 10 minutes, allowing the flavors to meld.

7. Serve the vegetarian lentil curry over a bed of cooked quinoa.

8. Garnish with fresh cilantro for a burst of freshness.

Mushroom and Spinach Stuffed Chicken Breast

Ingredients:

- 4 boneless, skinless chicken breasts
- 1 cup mushrooms, finely chopped

- 2 cups fresh spinach, chopped
- 1/2 cup feta cheese, crumbled
- 2 cloves garlic, minced
- 1 tablespoon olive oil
- 1 teaspoon dried oregano
- Salt and pepper to taste
- Toothpicks for securing

For Lemon Herb Sauce:

- Juice of 1 lemon
- 2 tablespoons olive oil
- 1 teaspoon dried thyme
- Salt and pepper to taste

Directions:

Stuffed Chicken:

1. Preheat the oven to 375°F (190°C).

2. In a skillet, heat olive oil over medium heat. Add chopped mushrooms and sauté until they release moisture and become golden brown.

3. Add minced garlic and chopped spinach to the skillet. Sauté until the spinach wilts.

4. Remove the skillet from heat and stir in crumbled feta cheese, dried oregano, salt, and pepper.

5. Butterfly each chicken breast by making a horizontal cut through the center, creating a pocket for the stuffing.

6. Stuff each chicken breast with the mushroom and spinach mixture and secure with toothpicks.

Baking:

1. Place the stuffed chicken breasts on a baking sheet.

2. Bake in the preheated oven for 25-30 minutes or until the chicken is cooked through and juices run clear.

Lemon Herb Sauce:

1. In a small bowl, whisk together lemon juice, olive oil, dried thyme, salt, and pepper.

Serving:

1. Remove toothpicks from the stuffed chicken breasts.

2. Drizzle the lemon herb sauce over the stuffed chicken before serving.

Baked Lemon Garlic Chicken with Roasted Vegetables

Ingredients:

For Chicken:

- 4 boneless, skinless chicken breasts
- 3 tablespoons olive oil
- Juice of 2 lemons
- 4 cloves garlic, minced
- 1 teaspoon dried thyme
- Salt and pepper to taste

For Roasted Vegetables:

- 2 cups baby potatoes, halved
- 2 cups baby carrots
- 1 zucchini, sliced
- 1 red bell pepper, sliced
- 1 tablespoon olive oil
- Salt and pepper to taste
- Fresh parsley for garnish

Directions:

Marinating Chicken:

1. In a bowl, mix olive oil, lemon juice, minced garlic, dried thyme, salt, and pepper.
2. Place chicken breasts in a resealable bag or shallow dish and pour the marinade over them.
3. Marinate in the refrigerator for at least 30 minutes, or preferably, overnight.

Baking Chicken:

1. Preheat the oven to 400°F (200°C).
2. Place marinated chicken breasts on a baking sheet.
3. Bake for 25-30 minutes or until the chicken is cooked through and juices run clear.

Roasting Vegetables:

1. In a separate baking dish, toss halved baby potatoes, baby carrots, sliced zucchini, and red bell pepper with olive oil, salt, and pepper.

2. Roast the vegetables in the oven for 20-25 minutes or until they are tender.

Serving:

1. Arrange the baked lemon garlic chicken on a serving plate.

2. Surround the chicken with the roasted vegetables.

3. Garnish with fresh parsley for added flavor.

Coconut Lime Shrimp Stir-Fry

Ingredients:

- 1 pound shrimp, peeled and deveined
- 2 tablespoons coconut oil
- 1 red bell pepper, thinly sliced
- 1 yellow bell pepper, thinly sliced
- 1 cup snap peas, ends trimmed
- 1 carrot, julienned
- 3 green onions, sliced
- 1 tablespoon fresh ginger, minced
- 2 cloves garlic, minced
- Zest and juice of 2 limes

- 1 can (14 oz) coconut milk
- 2 tablespoons soy sauce (low sodium)
- 1 tablespoon honey or maple syrup
- Salt and pepper to taste
- Fresh cilantro for garnish
- Cooked brown rice for serving

Directions:

Stir-Fry:

1. In a large wok or skillet, heat coconut oil over medium-high heat.
2. Add shrimp and cook until they turn pink and opaque. Remove shrimp from the wok and set aside.
3. In the same wok, add more coconut oil if needed. Sauté sliced bell peppers, snap peas, julienned carrot, green onions, minced ginger, and minced garlic for 3-4 minutes until vegetables are crisp-tender.

Coconut Lime Sauce:

1. In a bowl, whisk together lime zest, lime juice, coconut milk, soy sauce, honey or maple syrup, salt, and pepper.
2. Pour the coconut lime sauce over the vegetables in the wok.

Combining:

1. Add the cooked shrimp back into the wok and toss everything together until well coated.

2. Cook for an additional 2-3 minutes until heated through.

Serving:

1. Serve the Coconut Lime Shrimp Stir-Fry over cooked brown rice.

2. Garnish with fresh cilantro for a burst of flavor.

Herb-Crusted Baked Salmon with Quinoa and Asparagus

Ingredients:

For Salmon:

- 4 salmon filets
- 2 tablespoons Dijon mustard
- 1 tablespoon olive oil
- 1 tablespoon fresh dill, chopped
- 1 tablespoon fresh parsley, chopped
- 1 teaspoon lemon zest
- Salt and pepper to taste

For Quinoa and Asparagus:

- 1 cup quinoa, rinsed
- 2 cups vegetable broth or water
- 1 bunch asparagus, trimmed and halved
- 2 tablespoons olive oil
- 1 clove garlic, minced
- Salt and pepper to taste

Directions:

Herb-Crusted Baked Salmon:

1. Preheat the oven to 400°F (200°C).

2. In a bowl, mix Dijon mustard, olive oil, chopped dill, chopped parsley, lemon zest, salt, and pepper.

3. Place salmon fillets on a baking sheet and spread the herb mixture over each fillet.

4. Bake in the preheated oven for 12-15 minutes or until the salmon is cooked through and flakes easily.

Quinoa and Asparagus:

1. In a saucepan, combine quinoa and vegetable broth or water. Bring to a boil, then reduce heat to low, cover, and simmer for 15-20 minutes or until quinoa is cooked and the liquid is absorbed.

2. In a skillet, heat olive oil over medium heat. Add minced garlic and sauté for 1-2 minutes.

3. Add halved asparagus to the skillet and sauté until tender-crisp.

4. Stir in cooked quinoa and toss everything together. Season with salt and pepper.

Serving:

1. Plate the herb-crusted baked salmon on top of a bed of quinoa and asparagus.

2. Garnish with additional fresh herbs and a squeeze of lemon if desired.

Mango Avocado Chicken Salad

Ingredients:

For Grilled Chicken:

- 4 boneless, skinless chicken breasts
- 2 tablespoons olive oil
- 1 teaspoon ground cumin
- 1 teaspoon paprika
- Salt and pepper to taste

For Salad:

- 4 cups mixed salad greens
- 1 mango, peeled, pitted, and diced
- 1 avocado, peeled, pitted, and sliced
- 1 cucumber, thinly sliced
- 1/2 red onion, thinly sliced
- 1/4 cup fresh cilantro, chopped

For Lime Vinaigrette:

- Juice of 2 limes
- 3 tablespoons olive oil
- 1 teaspoon honey or maple syrup
- Salt and pepper to taste

Directions:

Grilled Chicken:

1. Preheat the grill or grill pan over medium-high heat.
2. In a bowl, mix olive oil, ground cumin, paprika, salt, and pepper.
3. Brush the chicken breasts with the spice mixture.
4. Grill the chicken for 6-8 minutes per side or until fully cooked.

Salad:

1. In a large salad bowl, combine mixed greens, diced mango, sliced avocado, cucumber, red onion, and chopped cilantro.

Lime Vinaigrette:

1. In a small bowl, whisk together lime juice, olive oil, honey or maple syrup, salt, and pepper.

Serving:

1. Slice the grilled chicken and place it on top of the salad.
2. Drizzle the lime vinaigrette over the salad.
3. Toss everything together gently.
4. Serve the Mango Avocado Chicken Salad for a refreshing and nutritious dinner.

Turmeric Ginger Lentil Stew with Spinach

Ingredients:

- 1 cup dry red lentils, rinsed
- 1 onion, finely chopped
- 3 cloves garlic, minced
- 1 tablespoon fresh ginger, grated
- 1 teaspoon ground turmeric
- 1 teaspoon ground cumin
- 1 teaspoon ground coriander
- 1/2 teaspoon cinnamon
- 4 cups vegetable broth
- 1 can (14 oz) diced tomatoes
- 3 carrots, peeled and diced
- 2 cups fresh spinach, chopped
- 2 tablespoons olive oil
- Salt and pepper to taste
- Fresh cilantro for garnish

Directions:

1. In a large pot, heat olive oil over medium heat. Add chopped onion and sauté until translucent.

2. Add minced garlic and grated ginger, continue sautéing for 1-2 minutes until fragrant.

3. Stir in ground turmeric, cumin, coriander, and cinnamon, coating the onions and garlic with the spices.

4. Add rinsed red lentils, diced tomatoes, diced carrots, and vegetable broth to the pot.

5. Bring the mixture to a boil, then reduce the heat to low, cover, and simmer for 20-25 minutes or until lentils are tender.

6. Stir in chopped fresh spinach and cook for an additional 5 minutes until the spinach wilts.

7. Season the stew with salt and pepper to taste.

Serving:

1. Ladle the turmeric ginger lentil stew into bowls.

2. Garnish with fresh cilantro for added flavor.

Sesame Garlic Tofu Stir-Fry with Broccoli and Brown Rice

Ingredients:

For Tofu:

- 1 block extra-firm tofu, pressed and cubed
- 3 tablespoons soy sauce (low sodium)
- 1 tablespoon sesame oil
- 1 tablespoon rice vinegar
- 2 teaspoons maple syrup or agave nectar
- 2 cloves garlic, minced
- 1 teaspoon grated ginger
- 1 tablespoon cornstarch

For Stir-Fry:

- 2 cups broccoli florets
- 1 red bell pepper, thinly sliced
- 1 carrot, julienned
- 2 cups cooked brown rice
- 2 tablespoons sesame seeds
- 2 green onions, sliced
- 2 tablespoons vegetable oil for cooking

Directions:

Tofu Preparation:

1. In a bowl, whisk together soy sauce, sesame oil, rice vinegar, maple syrup, minced garlic, and grated ginger.
2. Toss cubed tofu in the marinade and let it sit for at least 15 minutes.
3. Sprinkle cornstarch over the marinated tofu and toss to coat.

Stir-Frying:

1. Heat vegetable oil in a large skillet or wok over medium-high heat.
2. Add tofu to the skillet and cook until all sides are golden brown.
3. Remove the tofu from the skillet and set it aside.

4. In the same skillet, add more oil if needed. Stir-fry broccoli, red bell pepper, and julienned carrot until they are tender-crisp.

5. Add the cooked tofu back to the skillet and toss everything together.

Serving:

1. Serve the sesame garlic tofu stir-fry over cooked brown rice.

2. Garnish with sesame seeds and sliced green onions for added flavor.

Lemon Garlic Shrimp with Zucchini Noodles

Ingredients:

- 1 pound shrimp, peeled and deveined
- 4 medium zucchinis, spiralized into noodles
- 3 tablespoons olive oil
- 4 cloves garlic, minced
- Juice of 2 lemons
- 1 teaspoon lemon zest
- 1 teaspoon dried oregano
- Salt and pepper to taste
- Crushed red pepper flakes (optional for heat)
- Fresh parsley for garnish

Directions:

Zucchini Noodles:

1. Spiralize the zucchinis into noodles using a spiralizer.

2. Heat 2 tablespoons of olive oil in a large skillet over medium heat.

3. Add zucchini noodles and sauté for 2-3 minutes until just tender. Set aside.

Lemon Garlic Shrimp:

1. In the same skillet, add the remaining olive oil.

2. Add minced garlic and sauté for 1-2 minutes until fragrant.

3. Add shrimp to the skillet and cook for 2-3 minutes per side until they turn pink and opaque.

4. Pour lemon juice over the shrimp, add lemon zest, dried oregano, salt, pepper, and optional crushed red pepper flakes. Stir to combine.

Serving:

1. Place a portion of zucchini noodles on a plate.

2. Top with lemon garlic shrimp.

3. Garnish with fresh parsley.

Mushroom and Spinach Quinoa Risotto

Ingredients:

- 1 cup quinoa, rinsed

- 2 tablespoons olive oil
- 1 onion, finely chopped
- 2 cloves garlic, minced
- 8 oz mushrooms, sliced
- 4 cups fresh spinach, chopped
- 1 cup vegetable broth
- 1 cup low-fat milk or plant-based milk
- 1/2 cup grated Parmesan cheese
- Salt and pepper to taste
- Fresh parsley for garnish

Directions:

Quinoa:

1. In a saucepan, combine quinoa and vegetable broth. Bring to a boil, then reduce heat to low, cover, and simmer for 15-20 minutes or until quinoa is cooked and the liquid is absorbed.

Mushroom and Spinach Mixture:

1. In a large skillet, heat olive oil over medium heat.
2. Add chopped onion and sauté until translucent.
3. Add minced garlic and sliced mushrooms, cook until mushrooms are tender.
4. Stir in chopped spinach and cook until wilted.

Combining:

1. Add cooked quinoa to the skillet with the mushroom and spinach mixture.
2. Pour in the milk and stir until well combined.
3. Stir in grated Parmesan cheese until melted and the risotto has a creamy consistency.
4. Season with salt and pepper to taste.

Serving:

1. Spoon the Mushroom and Spinach Quinoa Risotto onto plates.
2. Garnish with fresh parsley.

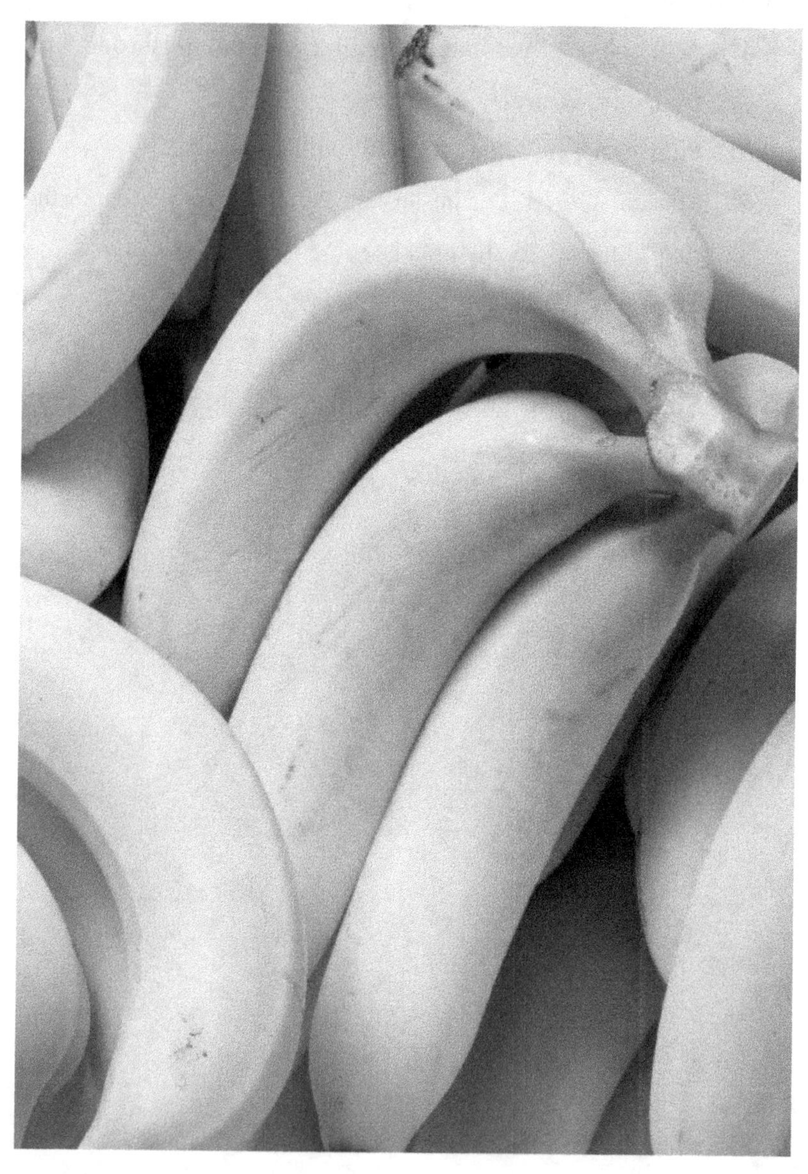

CHAPTER 7: SATISFYING SOUPS AND STEWS

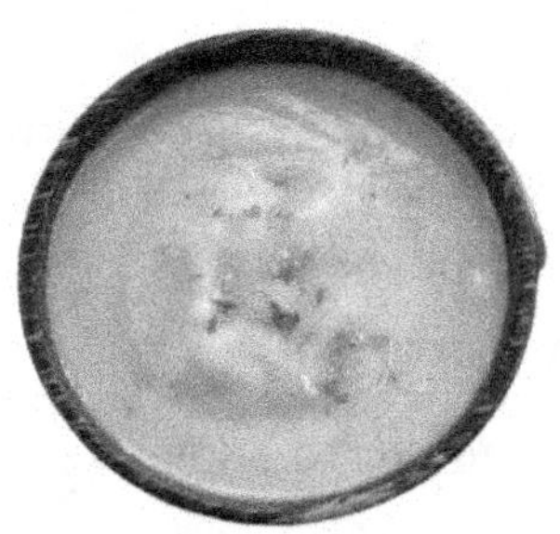

Lentil and Vegetable Soup

Ingredients:

- 1 cup dry green or brown lentils, rinsed
- 1 large carrot, diced
- 1 celery stalk, diced
- 1 onion, finely chopped
- 3 cloves garlic, minced
- 1 can (14 oz) diced tomatoes, undrained
- 6 cups low-sodium vegetable broth
- 1 teaspoon ground cumin
- 1 teaspoon ground coriander
- 1/2 teaspoon smoked paprika
- 1 bay leaf
- Salt and pepper to taste

- 2 cups chopped kale or spinach

- Juice of 1 lemon

- Fresh parsley for garnish (optional)

Directions:

1. Saute Vegetables:

   - In a large pot, sauté diced carrot, celery, and onion in a bit of olive oil over medium heat until softened.

2. Add Lentils and Spices:

   - Add rinsed lentils, minced garlic, ground cumin, ground coriander, smoked paprika, and the bay leaf to the pot. Stir well to coat the vegetables.

3. Pour Broth and Tomatoes:

   - Pour in the vegetable broth and add the undrained diced tomatoes. Bring the mixture to a boil.

4. Simmer:

   - Reduce heat, cover, and simmer for about 25-30 minutes or until the lentils are tender.

5. Season and Add Greens:

   - Season the soup with salt and pepper to taste. Stir in chopped kale or spinach and let it simmer for an additional 5 minutes until the greens are wilted.

6. Finish with Lemon Juice:
   - Remove the bay leaf and stir in the juice of one lemon.

7. Garnish and Serve:
   - Garnish with fresh parsley if desired.
   - Serve this Lentil and Vegetable Soup hot, providing a nutritious and comforting option.

Chickpea and Sweet Potato Stew

Ingredients:

- 2 cans (15 oz each) chickpeas, drained and rinsed
- 2 medium sweet potatoes, peeled and diced
- 1 onion, finely chopped
- 3 cloves garlic, minced
- 1 can (14 oz) diced tomatoes, undrained
- 4 cups low-sodium vegetable broth
- 1 teaspoon ground turmeric
- 1 teaspoon ground cumin
- 1/2 teaspoon ground cinnamon
- 1/2 teaspoon smoked paprika
- Salt and pepper to taste
- 2 cups chopped kale or spinach
- Juice of 1 lime
- Fresh cilantro for garnish (optional)

Directions:

1. Saute Onion and Garlic:

   o   In a large pot, sauté finely chopped onion and minced garlic in a bit of olive oil over medium heat until softened.

2. Add Sweet Potatoes and Spices:

   o   Add diced sweet potatoes, ground turmeric, ground cumin, ground cinnamon, and smoked paprika to the pot. Stir well to coat the vegetables in the spices.

3. Pour Broth and Tomatoes:

   o   Pour in the vegetable broth and add the undrained diced tomatoes. Bring the mixture to a simmer.

4. Cook Sweet Potatoes:

   o   Cover the pot and let it simmer for about 15-20 minutes or until the sweet potatoes are fork-tender.

5. Add Chickpeas and Greens:

   o   Stir in the drained and rinsed chickpeas along with chopped kale or spinach. Let it simmer for an additional 5-7 minutes until the greens are wilted.

6. Season and Finish with Lime Juice:

   o Season the stew with salt and pepper to taste. Squeeze the juice of one lime into the pot and stir.

7. Garnish and Serve:

   o Garnish with fresh cilantro if desired.

   o Serve this Chickpea and Sweet Potato Stew hot, offering a hearty and nutrient-rich option.

Broccoli and White Bean Soup

Ingredients:

- 1 large head of broccoli, florets separated and stems chopped
- 1 can (15 oz) white beans, drained and rinsed
- 1 onion, finely chopped
- 2 cloves garlic, minced
- 4 cups low-sodium vegetable broth
- 2 tablespoons olive oil
- 1 teaspoon dried thyme
- 1/2 teaspoon ground coriander
- Salt and pepper to taste
- 1 tablespoon lemon juice
- Optional: Grated Parmesan cheese for garnish

Directions:

1. Saute Onion and Garlic:
   - In a large pot, sauté finely chopped onion and minced garlic in olive oil over medium heat until softened.

2. Add Broccoli and Spices:
   - Add broccoli florets, chopped broccoli stems, dried thyme, and ground coriander to the pot. Stir to coat the vegetables in the spices.

3. Pour Broth and Simmer:
   - Pour in the vegetable broth, bring to a simmer, and cook for about 10-15 minutes or until the broccoli is tender.

4. Blend the Soup:
   - Use an immersion blender to blend the soup until smooth. Alternatively, transfer small batches to a blender and blend until smooth, then return to the pot.

5. Add White Beans:
   - Stir in the drained and rinsed white beans and let the soup simmer for an additional 5-7 minutes.

6. Season and Finish with Lemon Juice:
   - Season the soup with salt and pepper to taste. Add lemon juice and stir well.

7. Garnish and Serve:

    o Optional: Garnish with grated Parmesan cheese.

    o Serve this Broccoli and White Bean Soup hot, providing a nutritious and comforting option.

Turkey and Vegetable Quinoa Stew

Ingredients:

- 1 lb ground turkey
- 1 cup quinoa, rinsed
- 1 onion, finely chopped
- 2 carrots, peeled and diced
- 2 celery stalks, diced
- 3 cloves garlic, minced
- 1 can (14 oz) diced tomatoes, undrained
- 6 cups low-sodium chicken or vegetable broth
- 1 teaspoon dried thyme
- 1/2 teaspoon ground turmeric
- Salt and pepper to taste
- 2 cups chopped kale or spinach
- Juice of 1 lemon
- Fresh parsley for garnish (optional)

Directions:

1. Cook Turkey:

    o   In a large pot, cook the ground turkey over medium heat until browned. Break it into small pieces as it cooks.

2. Saute Vegetables:

    o   Add chopped onion, diced carrots, diced celery, and minced garlic to the pot. Saute until the vegetables are softened.

3. Add Quinoa and Spices:

    o   Stir in rinsed quinoa, dried thyme, ground turmeric, salt, and pepper. Cook for an additional 2-3 minutes.

4. Pour Broth and Tomatoes:

    o   Pour in the chicken or vegetable broth and add the undrained diced tomatoes. Bring the stew to a boil.

5. Simmer:

    o   Reduce heat, cover, and simmer for about 15-20 minutes or until the quinoa is cooked and the vegetables are tender.

6. Add Greens and Lemon Juice:

    o   Stir in chopped kale or spinach and let it simmer for an additional 5 minutes until the greens are wilted. Squeeze in the juice of one lemon.

7. Garnish and Serve:

    o   Optional: Garnish with fresh parsley.

    o   Serve this Turkey and Vegetable Quinoa Stew hot, offering a protein-packed and wholesome option.

Spinach and Chickpea Soup

Ingredients:

- 1 can (15 oz) chickpeas, drained and rinsed
- 4 cups fresh spinach, chopped
- 1 onion, finely chopped
- 2 carrots, peeled and diced
- 2 cloves garlic, minced
- 6 cups low-sodium vegetable broth
- 2 tablespoons olive oil
- 1 teaspoon ground cumin
- 1/2 teaspoon ground coriander
- 1/2 teaspoon dried oregano
- Salt and pepper to taste
- Juice of 1 lemon

- Fresh parsley for garnish (optional)

Directions:

1. Saute Onion and Garlic:
   - In a large pot, sauté finely chopped onion and minced garlic in olive oil over medium heat until softened.
2. Add Carrots and Spices:
   - Add diced carrots, ground cumin, ground coriander, and dried oregano to the pot. Stir to coat the vegetables in the spices.
3. Pour Broth and Chickpeas:
   - Pour in the vegetable broth and add the drained and rinsed chickpeas. Bring the mixture to a simmer.
4. Simmer:
   - Cover the pot and let it simmer for about 15-20 minutes or until the carrots are tender.
5. Add Spinach and Lemon Juice:
   - Stir in the chopped fresh spinach and let it simmer for an additional 5 minutes until the spinach is wilted. Squeeze in the juice of one lemon.

6. Season and Serve:

  - Season the soup with salt and pepper to taste.

  - Optional: Garnish with fresh parsley.

  - Serve this Spinach and Chickpea Soup hot, providing a nutrient-rich and flavorful option.

Mushroom and Quinoa Stew

Ingredients:

- 1 cup quinoa, rinsed
- 8 oz mushrooms, sliced (button mushrooms or your preferred variety)
- 1 onion, finely chopped
- 2 carrots, peeled and diced
- 3 cloves garlic, minced
- 4 cups low-sodium vegetable broth
- 2 tablespoons tomato paste
- 1 teaspoon dried thyme
- 1/2 teaspoon smoked paprika
- Salt and pepper to taste
- 1 cup chopped kale or spinach
- 2 tablespoons olive oil
- Fresh parsley for garnish (optional)

Directions:

1. Saute Vegetables:
   - In a large pot, sauté finely chopped onion and minced garlic in olive oil over medium heat until softened.
2. Add Mushrooms and Carrots:
   - Add sliced mushrooms and diced carrots to the pot. Cook for about 5 minutes until the mushrooms release their moisture.
3. Stir in Quinoa and Spices:
   - Stir in rinsed quinoa, dried thyme, smoked paprika, salt, and pepper. Cook for an additional 2-3 minutes.
4. Dissolve Tomato Paste:
   - Dissolve tomato paste in the vegetable broth and pour it into the pot.
5. Simmer:
   - Bring the stew to a simmer, cover, and let it cook for about 15-20 minutes or until the quinoa is cooked, and the vegetables are tender.
6. Add Greens:
   - Stir in chopped kale or spinach and let it simmer for an additional 5 minutes until the greens are wilted.

7. Season and Serve:

   o Adjust the seasoning if needed.

   o Optional: Garnish with fresh parsley.

   o Serve this Mushroom and Quinoa Stew hot, providing a hearty and wholesome option.

Sweet Potato and Lentil Soup

Ingredients:

- 1 cup dried red lentils, rinsed
- 2 medium-sized sweet potatoes, peeled and diced
- 1 onion, finely chopped
- 2 carrots, peeled and sliced
- 3 cloves garlic, minced
- 6 cups low-sodium vegetable broth
- 1 teaspoon ground cumin
- 1/2 teaspoon ground cinnamon
- 1/2 teaspoon smoked paprika
- Salt and pepper to taste
- 2 tablespoons olive oil
- Juice of 1 lemon
- Fresh cilantro for garnish (optional)

Directions:

1. Saute Vegetables:

    o In a large pot, sauté finely chopped onion and minced garlic in olive oil over medium heat until softened.

2. Add Sweet Potatoes and Carrots:

    o Add diced sweet potatoes and sliced carrots to the pot. Cook for about 5 minutes until they begin to soften.

3. Stir in Lentils and Spices:

    o Stir in rinsed red lentils, ground cumin, ground cinnamon, smoked paprika, salt, and pepper. Cook for an additional 2-3 minutes.

4. Pour in Broth:

    o Pour in the vegetable broth and bring the mixture to a boil.

5. Simmer:

    o Reduce heat, cover, and let it simmer for about 15-20 minutes or until the lentils are cooked, and the vegetables are tender.

6. Blend (Optional):

    o For a creamier texture, use an immersion blender to partially blend the soup. Leave some chunks for texture.

7. Finish with Lemon Juice:

   o Squeeze in the juice of one lemon and stir well.

8. Season and Serve:

   o Adjust the seasoning if needed.

   o Optional: Garnish with fresh cilantro.

   o Serve this Sweet Potato and Lentil Soup hot, offering a nutritious and flavorful option.

Chickpea and Vegetable Stew

Ingredients:

- 2 cans (15 oz each) chickpeas, drained and rinsed
- 2 zucchinis, diced
- 1 bell pepper, chopped (any color)
- 1 onion, finely chopped
- 3 cloves garlic, minced
- 4 cups low-sodium vegetable broth
- 1 can (14 oz) diced tomatoes, undrained
- 2 teaspoons ground cumin
- 1 teaspoon ground coriander
- 1/2 teaspoon smoked paprika
- Salt and pepper to taste
- 2 tablespoons olive oil
- Fresh parsley for garnish (optional)

Directions:

1. Saute Vegetables:
    - In a large pot, sauté finely chopped onion and minced garlic in olive oil over medium heat until softened.
2. Add Bell Pepper and Zucchini:
    - Add chopped bell pepper and diced zucchinis to the pot. Cook for about 5 minutes until the vegetables begin to soften.
3. Stir in Chickpeas and Spices:
    - Stir in drained chickpeas, ground cumin, ground coriander, smoked paprika, salt, and pepper. Cook for an additional 2-3 minutes.
4. Pour in Broth and Tomatoes:
    - Pour in the vegetable broth and add the undrained diced tomatoes. Bring the stew to a simmer.
5. Simmer:
    - Reduce heat, cover, and let it simmer for about 15-20 minutes or until the vegetables are tender.
6. Adjust Seasoning:
    - Taste and adjust the seasoning if needed.

7. Serve:

- o Optional: Garnish with fresh parsley.
- o Serve this Chickpea and Vegetable Stew hot, providing a protein-packed and satisfying option.

Butternut Squash and Apple Soup

Ingredients:

- 1 medium-sized butternut squash, peeled, seeded, and diced
- 2 apples, peeled, cored, and chopped
- 1 onion, finely chopped
- 3 cloves garlic, minced
- 4 cups low-sodium vegetable broth
- 1 teaspoon ground ginger
- 1/2 teaspoon ground cinnamon
- 1/4 teaspoon nutmeg
- Salt and pepper to taste
- 2 tablespoons olive oil
- 1 cup unsweetened almond milk (or any plant-based milk)
- Pumpkin seeds for garnish (optional)

Directions:

1. Saute Aromatics:
   - In a large pot, sauté finely chopped onion and minced garlic in olive oil over medium heat until softened.
2. Add Butternut Squash and Apple:
   - Add diced butternut squash and chopped apples to the pot. Cook for about 5 minutes until they start to soften.
3. Stir in Spices:
   - Stir in ground ginger, ground cinnamon, nutmeg, salt, and pepper. Cook for an additional 2-3 minutes.
4. Pour in Broth:
   - Pour in the vegetable broth and bring the mixture to a boil.
5. Simmer:
   - Reduce heat, cover, and let it simmer for about 15-20 minutes or until the butternut squash is tender.
6. Blend:
   - Use an immersion blender to blend the soup until smooth. Alternatively, transfer the mixture to a blender and blend in batches.

7. Finish with Almond Milk:

    o   Stir in the almond milk to add creaminess to the
        soup.

8. Adjust Seasoning:

    o   Taste and adjust the seasoning if needed.

9. Serve:

    o   Optional: Garnish with pumpkin seeds.

    o   Serve this Butternut Squash and Apple Soup hot,
        offering a comforting and nutritious option.

Quinoa and Black Bean Stew

Ingredients:

- 1 cup quinoa, rinsed
- 2 cans (15 oz each) black beans, drained and rinsed
- 1 red bell pepper, diced
- 1 yellow bell pepper, diced
- 1 onion, finely chopped
- 3 cloves garlic, minced
- 4 cups low-sodium vegetable broth
- 1 can (14 oz) diced tomatoes, undrained
- 2 teaspoons ground cumin
- 1 teaspoon smoked paprika
- Salt and pepper to taste
- 2 tablespoons olive oil

- Fresh cilantro for garnish (optional)

Directions:

1. Saute Aromatics:
   - In a large pot, sauté finely chopped onion and minced garlic in olive oil over medium heat until softened.

2. Add Bell Peppers:
   - Add diced red and yellow bell peppers to the pot. Cook for about 5 minutes until the peppers begin to soften.

3. Stir in Quinoa and Spices:
   - Stir in rinsed quinoa, ground cumin, smoked paprika, salt, and pepper. Cook for an additional 2-3 minutes.

4. Pour in Broth and Tomatoes:
   - Pour in the vegetable broth and add the undrained diced tomatoes. Bring the stew to a simmer.

5. Simmer:
   - Reduce heat, cover, and let it simmer for about 15-20 minutes or until the quinoa is cooked and the vegetables are tender.

6. Add Black Beans:

   o Stir in drained and rinsed black beans. Cook for an additional 5 minutes to heat the beans through.

7. Adjust Seasoning:

   o Taste and adjust the seasoning if needed.

8. Serve:

   o Optional: Garnish with fresh cilantro.

   o Serve this Quinoa and Black Bean Stew hot, providing a protein-rich and flavorful option.

Spinach and White Bean Soup

Ingredients:

- 1 can (15 oz) white beans, drained and rinsed
- 4 cups fresh spinach, chopped
- 1 onion, finely chopped
- 2 carrots, peeled and sliced
- 3 cloves garlic, minced
- 4 cups low-sodium vegetable broth
- 1 teaspoon dried thyme
- 1/2 teaspoon dried rosemary
- 1/2 teaspoon onion powder
- Salt and pepper to taste
- 2 tablespoons olive oil

- Juice of 1 lemon
- Grated Parmesan cheese for garnish (optional)

Directions:

1. Saute Vegetables:
   - In a large pot, sauté finely chopped onion and minced garlic in olive oil over medium heat until softened.
2. Add Carrots and Beans:
   - Add sliced carrots and drained white beans to the pot. Cook for about 5 minutes until the carrots start to soften.
3. Stir in Herbs and Seasonings:
   - Stir in dried thyme, dried rosemary, onion powder, salt, and pepper. Cook for an additional 2-3 minutes.
4. Pour in Broth:
   - Pour in the vegetable broth and bring the mixture to a boil.
5. Simmer:
   - Reduce heat, cover, and let it simmer for about 15-20 minutes or until the vegetables are tender.
6. Add Spinach:
   - Stir in chopped fresh spinach and cook until wilted.

7. Finish with Lemon Juice:

    o   Squeeze in the juice of one lemon and stir well.

8. Adjust Seasoning:

    o   Taste and adjust the seasoning if needed.

9. Serve:

    o   Optional: Garnish with grated Parmesan cheese.

    o   Serve this Spinach and White Bean Soup hot, providing a nutrient-packed and comforting option.

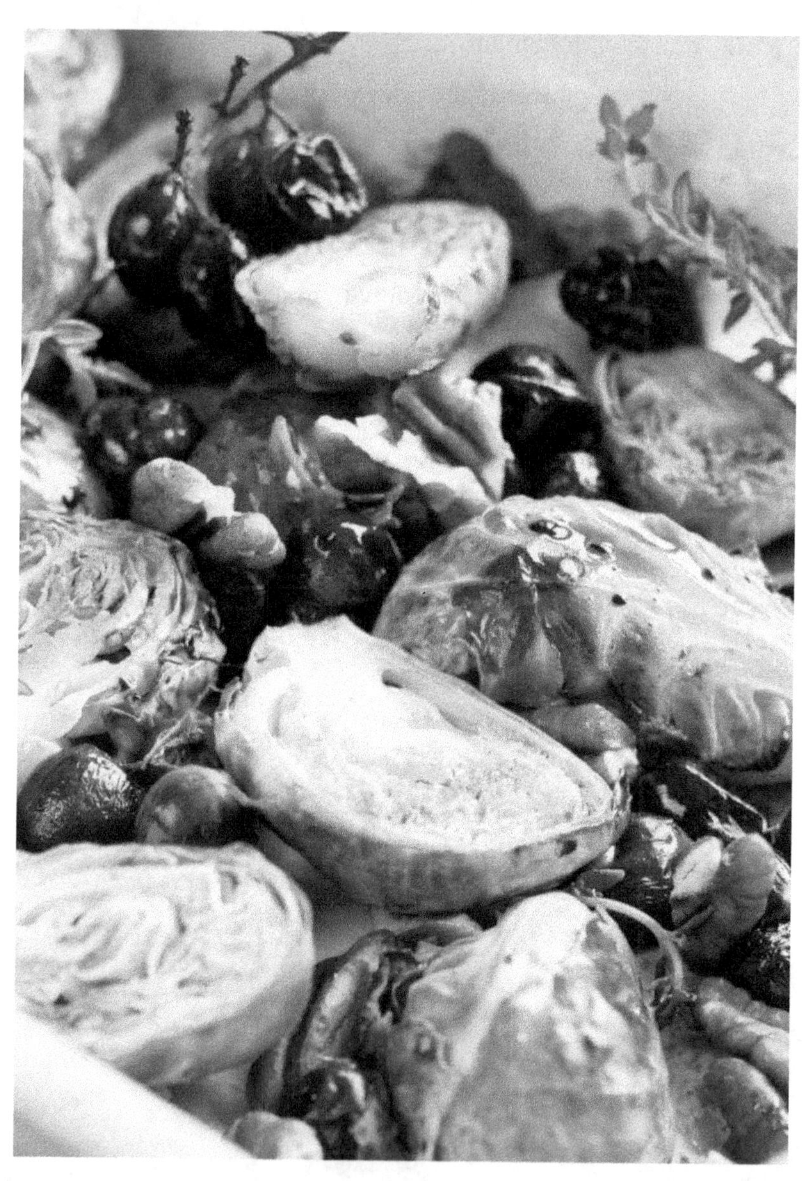

CHAPTER 8: VEGETABLE DISHES

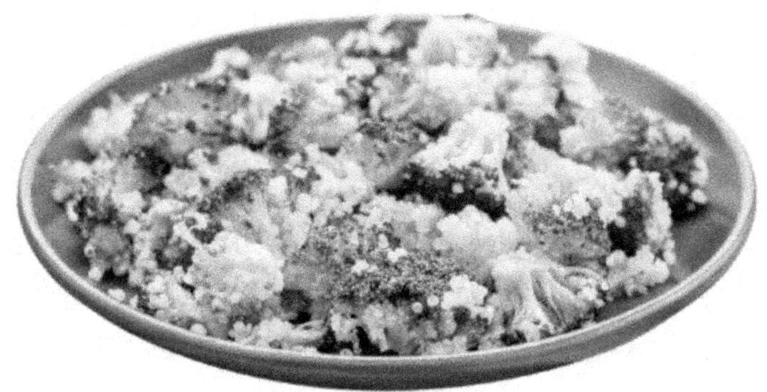

Garlic Roasted Broccoli and Carrots

Ingredients:

- 2 cups broccoli florets
- 2 cups baby carrots
- 3 tablespoons olive oil
- 3 cloves garlic, minced
- 1 teaspoon dried thyme
- 1 teaspoon paprika
- Salt and pepper to taste
- Lemon wedges for serving (optional)

Directions:

Preheat the Oven:

1. Preheat your oven to 425°F (220°C).

2. Prepare Vegetables:

   - Wash and trim the broccoli into bite-sized florets.
   - If using whole baby carrots, you can leave them as is or cut them into halves or quarters for quicker roasting.

3. Garlic Herb Oil:

   - In a small bowl, mix together olive oil, minced garlic, dried thyme, paprika, salt, and pepper.

4. Coat Vegetables:

   - Place broccoli florets and baby carrots in a large mixing bowl.
   - Pour the garlic herb oil over the vegetables and toss until they are evenly coated.

5. Roasting:

   - Spread the coated vegetables on a baking sheet in a single layer.
   - Roast in the preheated oven for 20-25 minutes or until the edges of the vegetables are golden brown and crispy.

6. Serve:

   - Remove from the oven and transfer to a serving dish.

o   Squeeze fresh lemon juice over the roasted broccoli and carrots for added flavor (optional).

o   Serve as a side dish alongside your protein of choice.

Lemon Herb Grilled Asparagus

Ingredients:

- 1 bunch fresh asparagus, trimmed
- 2 tablespoons olive oil
- Zest of 1 lemon
- Juice of 1 lemon
- 2 teaspoons dried oregano
- Salt and pepper to taste

Directions:

Preheat the Grill:

1.   Preheat your grill or grill pan over medium-high heat.
2.   Prepare Asparagus:

     o   Trim the tough ends of the asparagus spears.

     o   In a shallow dish, toss the asparagus with olive oil, lemon zest, lemon juice, dried oregano, salt, and pepper. Ensure the asparagus is evenly coated.

3. Grilling:

- o   Place the asparagus on the preheated grill, arranging them perpendicular to the grill grates to prevent them from falling through.
- o   Grill for 5-7 minutes, turning occasionally until the asparagus is tender and has a slight char.

4. Serve:

- o   Transfer the grilled asparagus to a serving platter.
- o   Drizzle any remaining lemon herb mixture over the asparagus.
- o   Serve immediately as a flavorful and nutritious side dish.

Honey Glazed Roasted Brussels Sprouts

Ingredients:

- 1 pound Brussels sprouts, trimmed and halved
- 2 tablespoons olive oil
- 2 tablespoons honey
- 1 tablespoon balsamic vinegar
- 1 teaspoon Dijon mustard
- Salt and pepper to taste
- Chopped fresh parsley for garnish (optional)

Directions:

Preheat the Oven:

1. Preheat your oven to 400°F (200°C).

2. Prepare Brussels Sprouts:

    o   Trim the tough ends of the Brussels sprouts and
        cut them in half.

    o   Place them in a large bowl.

3. Honey Glaze Mixture:

    o   In a small bowl, whisk together olive oil, honey,
        balsamic vinegar, Dijon mustard, salt, and
        pepper.

4. Coat Brussels Sprouts:

    o   Pour the honey glaze mixture over the Brussels
        sprouts and toss until they are evenly coated.

5. Roasting:

    o   Spread the coated Brussels sprouts on a baking
        sheet in a single layer.

    o   Roast in the preheated oven for 20-25 minutes or
        until they are golden brown and crisp on the
        edges.

6. Serve:

    o   Transfer the roasted Brussels sprouts to a
        serving dish.

    o   Garnish with chopped fresh parsley if desired.

Sesame Ginger Stir-Fried Vegetables

Ingredients:

- 2 cups broccoli florets
- 1 red bell pepper, thinly sliced
- 1 yellow bell pepper, thinly sliced
- 1 cup snap peas, ends trimmed
- 2 carrots, julienned
- 3 tablespoons low-sodium soy sauce
- 1 tablespoon sesame oil
- 1 tablespoon rice vinegar
- 1 tablespoon honey
- 1 tablespoon fresh ginger, grated
- 2 cloves garlic, minced
- 2 tablespoons sesame seeds
- 2 tablespoons green onions, chopped (for garnish)
- 2 tablespoons vegetable oil (for stir-frying)
- Cooked brown rice or quinoa (optional, for serving)

Directions:

1. Prepare Vegetables:
   - Cut broccoli into small florets.
   - Thinly slice red and yellow bell peppers.
   - Trim snap peas and julienne carrots.

2. Sauce Mixture:

   o In a small bowl, whisk together soy sauce, sesame oil, rice vinegar, honey, grated ginger, and minced garlic.

3. Stir-Frying:

   o Heat vegetable oil in a wok or large skillet over medium-high heat.

   o Add broccoli, bell peppers, snap peas, and carrots. Stir-fry for 4-5 minutes until the vegetables are crisp-tender.

4. Add Sauce:

   o Pour the sauce mixture over the stir-fried vegetables. Toss to coat evenly.

5. Finish and Serve:

   o Sprinkle sesame seeds over the vegetables and toss for an additional 1-2 minutes until everything is well combined.

   o Garnish with chopped green onions.

   o Serve over cooked brown rice or quinoa if desired.

Mediterranean Roasted Eggplant and Zucchini

Ingredients:

- 1 large eggplant, diced
- 2 medium zucchinis, sliced
- 1 red onion, thinly sliced
- 2 bell peppers (red or yellow), sliced
- 3 tablespoons olive oil
- 2 teaspoons dried oregano
- 1 teaspoon dried basil
- 1 teaspoon garlic powder
- Salt and pepper to taste
- 1 tablespoon balsamic vinegar
- Fresh parsley for garnish

Directions:

Preheat the Oven:

1. Preheat your oven to 400°F (200°C).
2. Prepare Vegetables:
   - Dice the eggplant, slice the zucchinis, thinly slice the red onion, and slice the bell peppers.

3. Roasting:

  - In a large mixing bowl, toss the diced eggplant, sliced zucchinis, red onion, and bell peppers with olive oil, dried oregano, dried basil, garlic powder, salt, and pepper.
  - Spread the seasoned vegetables on a baking sheet in a single layer.

4. Baking:

  - Roast in the preheated oven for 25-30 minutes, or until the vegetables are tender and lightly browned, tossing halfway through.

5. Finish and Serve:

  - Drizzle the roasted vegetables with balsamic vinegar and toss to combine.
  - Garnish with fresh parsley before serving.

Balsamic Glazed Roasted Vegetables

Ingredients:

- 2 cups baby carrots
- 1 medium zucchini, sliced
- 1 cup cherry tomatoes
- 1 red onion, cut into wedges
- 2 tablespoons olive oil
- 3 tablespoons balsamic vinegar

- 1 tablespoon honey

- 1 teaspoon dried thyme

- Salt and pepper to taste

- Chopped fresh basil for garnish (optional)

Directions:

Preheat the Oven:

1. Preheat your oven to 400°F (200°C).

2. Prepare Vegetables:

    o In a large bowl, toss baby carrots, zucchini slices, cherry tomatoes, and red onion wedges with olive oil.

3. Balsamic Glaze:

    o In a small bowl, whisk together balsamic vinegar, honey, dried thyme, salt, and pepper.

4. Coat Vegetables:

    o Pour the balsamic glaze over the vegetables and toss until they are evenly coated.

5. Roasting:

    o Spread the coated vegetables on a baking sheet in a single layer.

6. Bake:

    o Roast in the preheated oven for 20-25 minutes or until the vegetables are tender and caramelized, stirring halfway through.

7. Garnish and Serve:

    o Remove from the oven and garnish with chopped fresh basil if desired.

    o Serve these Balsamic Glazed Roasted Vegetables as a delicious and nutritious side dish.

Cauliflower and Broccoli Gratin

Ingredients:

- 1 head cauliflower, cut into florets
- 1 head broccoli, cut into florets
- 2 tablespoons olive oil
- 3 cloves garlic, minced
- 2 tablespoons whole wheat flour
- 2 cups low-fat milk
- 1 cup shredded sharp cheddar cheese
- 1/4 cup grated Parmesan cheese
- Salt and pepper to taste
- 1/2 teaspoon dried thyme
- 1/2 cup whole wheat breadcrumbs
- Fresh parsley for garnish (optional)

Directions:

Preheat the Oven:

1. Preheat your oven to 375°F (190°C).

2. Steam Vegetables:

  o Steam cauliflower and broccoli florets until they are just tender. Drain and set aside.

3. Prepare Cheese Sauce:

  o In a saucepan, heat olive oil over medium heat. Add minced garlic and cook until fragrant.

  o Stir in whole wheat flour and cook for 1-2 minutes.

  o Gradually whisk in low-fat milk, ensuring there are no lumps. Cook until the mixture thickens.

  o Reduce heat and add shredded cheddar and Parmesan cheeses. Stir until the cheese is melted and the sauce is smooth.

4. Season and Assemble:

  o Season the cheese sauce with salt, pepper, and dried thyme.

  o Combine the steamed cauliflower and broccoli with the cheese sauce, ensuring the vegetables are well coated.

5. Bake:

  o Transfer the mixture to a baking dish. Sprinkle whole wheat breadcrumbs over the top.

  o Bake in the preheated oven for 20-25 minutes or until the top is golden brown.

6. Garnish and Serve:

    o Garnish with fresh parsley if desired.

    o Serve this Cauliflower and Broccoli Gratin as a flavorful and satisfying vegetable dish.

Spaghetti Squash Primavera

Ingredients:

- 1 medium spaghetti squash
- 2 tablespoons olive oil
- 2 cloves garlic, minced
- 1 cup cherry tomatoes, halved
- 1 cup broccoli florets
- 1/2 cup sliced bell peppers (any color)
- 1/4 cup grated Parmesan cheese
- 2 tablespoons fresh basil, chopped
- Salt and pepper to taste
- Optional: Crushed red pepper flakes for a bit of heat

Directions:

1. Prepare Spaghetti Squash:

    o Preheat your oven to 400°F (200°C).

    o Cut the spaghetti squash in half lengthwise and remove the seeds.

- Place the halves on a baking sheet, cut side up. Drizzle with olive oil, sprinkle with salt and pepper.
    - Roast in the oven for 40-45 minutes or until the squash is tender.
2. Cook Vegetables:
    - In a large skillet, heat olive oil over medium heat. Add minced garlic and sauté for 1 minute.
    - Add cherry tomatoes, broccoli florets, and sliced bell peppers to the skillet. Cook until the vegetables are slightly tender but still vibrant.
3. Scrape Squash and Combine:
    - Once the spaghetti squash is done roasting, use a fork to scrape the flesh into "spaghetti" strands.
    - Add the spaghetti squash strands to the skillet with the sautéed vegetables. Toss everything together.
4. Season and Finish:
    - Season with salt, pepper, and optional crushed red pepper flakes for some heat.
    - Sprinkle grated Parmesan cheese over the mixture and toss until well combined.
    - Garnish with fresh chopped basil.
5. Serve and enjoy this Spaghetti Squash Primavera!

CHAPTER 9: NUTRIENT-PACKED SMOOTHIES

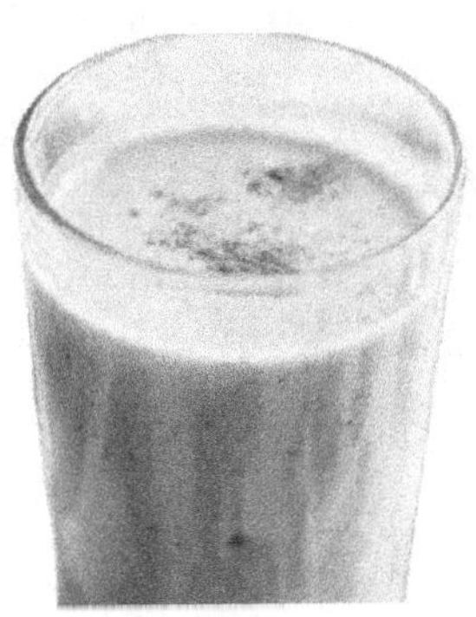

Green Berry Anti-Inflammatory Smoothie

Ingredients:

- 1 cup spinach leaves (fresh or frozen)
- 1/2 cup blueberries (fresh or frozen)
- 1/2 cup strawberries (fresh or frozen)
- 1/2 cucumber, peeled and sliced
- 1/2 avocado
- 1 tablespoon chia seeds
- 1 cup coconut water
- Ice cubes (optional for a colder texture)

Directions:

1. Place spinach, blueberries, strawberries, cucumber, avocado, and chia seeds in a blender.

2. Add coconut water to the blender for a hydrating base.

3. Blend on high speed until the mixture becomes smooth and creamy.

4. If you prefer a colder consistency, add ice cubes and blend again.

5. Pour the smoothie into a glass and enjoy this nutrient-packed, anti-inflammatory beverage.

Tropical Turmeric Boost Smoothie

Ingredients:

- 1 cup pineapple chunks (fresh or frozen)
- 1/2 banana
- 1/2 cup mango chunks (fresh or frozen)
- 1/2 teaspoon turmeric powder
- 1 tablespoon flaxseeds
- 1/2 cup Greek yogurt (or a dairy-free alternative)
- 1 cup almond milk
- Honey to taste (optional)

Directions:

1. Combine pineapple chunks, banana, mango chunks, turmeric powder, flaxseeds, Greek yogurt, and almond milk in a blender.

2. Blend on high speed until all ingredients are well combined and the mixture is smooth.

3. Taste the smoothie and add honey if desired for sweetness.

4. Pour the smoothie into a glass and savor the tropical flavors with the added benefits of turmeric and flaxseeds.

Berry Citrus Vitality Smoothie

Ingredients:

- 1 cup mixed berries (strawberries, blueberries, raspberries)
- 1/2 orange, peeled
- 1/2 cup cucumber, diced
- 1/2 cup kale leaves, stems removed
- 1 tablespoon hemp seeds
- 1/2 cup coconut water
- Ice cubes (optional)

Directions:

1. Place mixed berries, peeled orange, diced cucumber, kale leaves, and hemp seeds in a blender.

2. Add coconut water for a hydrating and nutrient-rich base.

3. Blend on high speed until the ingredients are well combined and the smoothie reaches a desired consistency.

4. If you prefer a colder texture, add ice cubes and blend again.

5. Pour the vibrant smoothie into a glass, and enjoy the refreshing and antioxidant-rich goodness.

Minty Green Immune Booster Smoothie

Ingredients:

- 1 cup spinach leaves (fresh or frozen)
- 1/2 green apple, cored and sliced
- 1/2 cup pineapple chunks (fresh or frozen)
- A handful of fresh mint leaves
- 1 tablespoon ginger, grated
- 1 tablespoon flaxseeds
- 1 cup coconut water or water
- Ice cubes (optional)

Directions:

1. Combine spinach leaves, green apple slices, pineapple chunks, fresh mint leaves, grated ginger, and flaxseeds in a blender.

2. Add coconut water or water for a refreshing liquid base.

3. Blend on high speed until the ingredients form a smooth and vibrant mixture.

4. If you prefer a colder consistency, include ice cubes and blend again.

5. Pour the invigorating smoothie into a glass, and relish the combination of greens, fruits, and herbs for a boost to your immune system.

Turmeric Mango Bliss Smoothie

Ingredients:

- 1 cup mango chunks (fresh or frozen)
- 1/2 banana
- 1/2 cup carrot juice
- 1/2 teaspoon turmeric powder
- 1 tablespoon almond butter
- 1/2 cup plain yogurt or dairy-free alternative
- 1 tablespoon honey (optional for added sweetness)
- 1/2 cup water or coconut water

Directions:

1. Combine mango chunks, banana, carrot juice, turmeric powder, almond butter, yogurt, and water in a blender.
2. Blend on high speed until the ingredients are well incorporated and the smoothie reaches a creamy consistency.
3. Taste the mixture and add honey if desired for additional sweetness.
4. Pour the golden-hued smoothie into a glass, savoring the tropical and anti-inflammatory flavors.

Peachy Green Energizer Smoothie

Ingredients:

- 1 cup frozen peach slices
- 1/2 cucumber, peeled and sliced
- 1/2 cup kale leaves, stems removed
- 1/2 cup plain kefir or yogurt (dairy or non-dairy)
- 1 tablespoon almond butter
- 1 teaspoon matcha powder
- 1 tablespoon honey (optional for sweetness)
- 1/2 cup water or coconut water

Directions:

1. Place frozen peach slices, cucumber, kale leaves, kefir or yogurt, almond butter, matcha powder, honey, and water in a blender.

2. Blend on high speed until the ingredients are well combined, and the smoothie achieves a velvety texture.

3. Taste the mixture and add honey if a touch of sweetness is desired.

4. Pour the Peachy Green Energizer Smoothie into a glass, relishing the delightful fusion of peachy goodness and the energy boost from matcha.

Cherry Almond Protein Power Smoothie

Ingredients:

- 1 cup cherries (fresh or frozen, pitted)
- 1/2 cup almond milk
- 1/2 cup Greek yogurt or plant-based yogurt
- 1 tablespoon almond butter
- 1 scoop protein powder (plant-based or whey, as per preference)
- 1 tablespoon honey (optional for sweetness)
- 1/2 teaspoon cinnamon
- Ice cubes (optional)

Directions:

1. Combine cherries, almond milk, Greek yogurt, almond butter, protein powder, honey, and cinnamon in a blender.

2. Blend on high speed until the ingredients are well combined, and the smoothie achieves a creamy texture.

3. If desired, add ice cubes for a colder consistency, then blend again.

4. Pour the Cherry Almond Protein Power Smoothie into a glass, enjoying the sweet and nutty flavors along with the protein boost.

Pomegranate Ginger Citrus Burst Smoothie

Ingredients:

- 1 cup pomegranate seeds
- 1/2 orange, peeled and segmented
- 1/2 lime, juiced
- 1/2 inch fresh ginger, peeled
- 1/2 cup plain kefir or yogurt (dairy or non-dairy)
- 1 tablespoon hemp seeds
- 1 tablespoon honey (optional for sweetness)
- 1/2 cup water or coconut water

Directions:

1. Combine pomegranate seeds, orange segments, lime juice, fresh ginger, kefir or yogurt, hemp seeds, honey, and water in a blender.
2. Blend on high speed until the ingredients are well combined, and the smoothie achieves a vibrant and zesty texture.
3. Adjust sweetness by adding honey if desired.
4. Pour the Pomegranate Ginger Citrus Burst Smoothie into a glass, savoring the burst of flavors and the immune-boosting properties.

Kiwi Basil Bliss Smoothie

Ingredients:

- 2 kiwis, peeled and sliced
- 1/2 cup fresh pineapple chunks
- 1/2 cup cucumber, diced
- 1/2 cup coconut water
- 1 tablespoon fresh basil leaves
- 1 tablespoon chia seeds
- 1/2 lemon, juiced
- Ice cubes (optional)

Directions:

1. Combine kiwi slices, pineapple chunks, cucumber, coconut water, fresh basil leaves, chia seeds, and lemon juice in a blender.

2. Blend on high speed until the ingredients are well combined, and the smoothie reaches a refreshing consistency.

3. Add ice cubes if you prefer a colder texture, then blend again.

4. Pour the Kiwi Basil Bliss Smoothie into a glass, enjoying the unique combination of kiwi, pineapple, and the subtle herbaceous notes from basil.

Mango Mint Hydration Elixir

Ingredients:

- 1 cup mango chunks (fresh or frozen)
- 1/2 cup cucumber, peeled and sliced
- 1/2 cup fresh mint leaves
- 1/2 lime, juiced
- 1/2 teaspoon spirulina powder (optional for added nutrients)
- 1 tablespoon pumpkin seeds
- 1/2 cup coconut water
- Ice cubes (optional)

Directions:

1. Combine mango chunks, cucumber, fresh mint leaves, lime juice, spirulina powder (if using), pumpkin seeds, and coconut water in a blender.
2. Blend on high speed until the ingredients are well combined, and the smoothie reaches a refreshing and vibrant texture.
3. Add ice cubes if you prefer a colder consistency, then blend again.
4. Pour the Mango Mint Hydration Elixir into a glass, savoring the tropical sweetness, cooling mint, and hydrating coconut water.

Blueberry Avocado Protein Boost Smoothie

Ingredients:

- 1 cup blueberries (fresh or frozen)
- 1/2 ripe avocado
- 1/2 cup spinach leaves (fresh or frozen)
- 1 scoop protein powder (plant-based or whey, as per preference)
- 1 tablespoon almond butter
- 1/2 cup almond milk
- 1 tablespoon chia seeds
- Ice cubes (optional)

Directions:

1. Combine blueberries, ripe avocado, spinach leaves, protein powder, almond butter, almond milk, and chia seeds in a blender.
2. Blend on high speed until the ingredients are well combined, and the smoothie reaches a creamy and nutrient-packed texture.
3. Add ice cubes if you prefer a colder consistency, then blend again.
4. Pour the Blueberry Avocado Protein Boost Smoothie into a glass, enjoying the antioxidant-rich blueberries and the creamy texture from avocado.

Raspberry Coconut Lime Refresher

Ingredients:

- 1 cup raspberries (fresh or frozen)
- 1/2 cup coconut milk
- 1/2 lime, juiced
- 1/2 cup zucchini, sliced
- 1 tablespoon shredded coconut
- 1 tablespoon hemp seeds
- 1 tablespoon honey (optional for sweetness)
- Ice cubes (optional)

Directions:

1. Combine raspberries, coconut milk, lime juice, zucchini, shredded coconut, hemp seeds, and honey (if using) in a blender.

2. Blend on high speed until the ingredients are well combined, and the smoothie reaches a refreshing and tangy texture.

3. If you prefer a colder consistency, add ice cubes and blend again.

4. Pour the Raspberry Coconut Lime Refresher into a glass, savoring the delightful combination of raspberry tartness and tropical coconut.

Peach Turmeric Zing Smoothie

Ingredients:

- 1 cup peach slices (fresh or frozen)
- 1/2 teaspoon turmeric powder
- 1/2 cup carrots, diced
- 1/2 cup unsweetened almond milk
- 1 tablespoon walnuts
- 1/2 teaspoon cinnamon
- 1/2 cup plain kefir or yogurt (dairy or non-dairy)
- Ice cubes (optional)

Directions:

1. Combine peach slices, turmeric powder, diced carrots, almond milk, walnuts, cinnamon, and kefir or yogurt in a blender.
2. Blend on high speed until the ingredients are well combined, and the smoothie achieves a smooth and velvety texture.
3. Add ice cubes if you prefer a colder consistency, then blend again.
4. Pour the Peach Turmeric Zing Smoothie into a glass, enjoying the peachy sweetness with a hint of turmeric and nutty undertones.

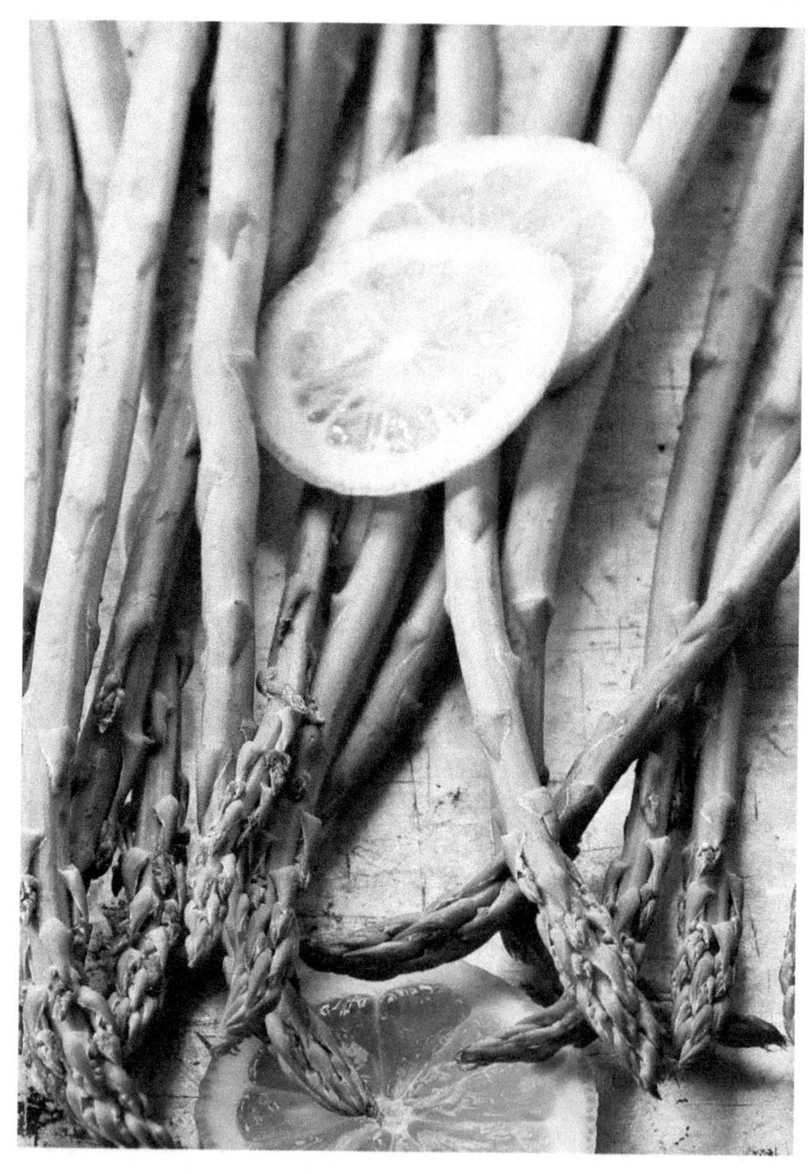

CONCLUSION

As you reach the end of this culinary guide for persons dealing with non-Hodgkin lymphoma, we hope you find inspiration and empowerment in the kitchen. The Non-Hodgkin Lymphoma Cookbook is more than simply a collection of dishes, it's a guide on your path to recovery and wellbeing.

You have in your hands a carefully developed resource that includes recipes specifically tailored to promote your health during and after treatment. Each meal is a representation of food's healing power, containing cancer-fighting nutrients with anti-inflammatory effects.

By incorporating nutrient-dense foods, lean meats, and a range of colorful fruits and vegetables, you are not only producing meals but also laying the groundwork for resilience. The cookbook demonstrates the view that a well-balanced, tasty food may be a valuable ally in the battle against Non-Hodgkin Lymphoma.

In the world of cancer-fighting foods, our recipes stress both taste and the science behind each item. Turmeric and ginger have anti-inflammatory properties, while a variety of fruits and vegetables provide critical vitamins and antioxidants.

Lean proteins help to maintain muscle mass and strengthen the immune system.

Remember that you are not alone as you browse these pages for recipes. This cookbook complements your medical therapy by providing you with a tool for managing your nutritional well-being. It is a celebration of the art and joy of cooking, transforming the kitchen into a therapeutic and nourishing environment.

Whether you're looking for comfort in a cup of anti-inflammatory soup, appreciating the brilliant tastes of a nutrient-dense salad, or experiencing the satisfaction of a nutritious, well-balanced dinner, each recipe adds to your overall health. Your journey is unique, and so should your diet be.

Allow this Non-Hodgkin Lymphoma Cookbook to assist you on this gastronomic trip, since it provides not just dishes but also a road map to resistance. Here's to food, strength, and an unyielding spirit that will carry you through your recovery. May these dishes bring you peace, pleasure, and the nourishment you need to thrive on your road beyond Non-Hodgkin Lymphoma.

NON-HODGKIN LYMPHOMA DIET
WEEKLY MEAL PLAN

Weekly
Meal Plan

Week: _______________

	BREAKFAST	LUNCH	DINNER	SNACKS
MON				
TUE				
WED				
THU				
FRI				
SAT				
SUN				

Shopping list

_______________ _______________

_______________ _______________

_______________ _______________

Notes:

Weekly
Meal Plan

Week: _____________

	BREAKFAST	LUNCH	DINNER	SNACKS
MON				
TUE				
WED				
THU				
FRI				
SAT				
SUN				

Shopping list

___________ ___________

___________ ___________

___________ ___________

Notes:

Weekly
Meal Plan

Week: _______________

	BREAKFAST	LUNCH	DINNER	SNACKS
MON				
TUE				
WED				
THU				
FRI				
SAT				
SUN				

Shopping list

_______________ _______________

_______________ _______________

_______________ _______________

Notes:

Weekly
Meal Plan

Week: _______________

	BREAKFAST	LUNCH	DINNER	SNACKS
MON				
TUE				
WED				
THU				
FRI				
SAT				
SUN				

Shopping list

_______________ _______________

_______________ _______________

_______________ _______________

Notes:

Weekly
Meal Plan

Week: _______________

	BREAKFAST	LUNCH	DINNER	SNACKS
MON				
TUE				
WED				
THU				
FRI				
SAT				
SUN				

Shopping list

_____________ _____________

_____________ _____________

_____________ _____________

Notes:

Weekly
Meal Plan

Week: ___________

	BREAKFAST	LUNCH	DINNER	SNACKS
MON				
TUE				
WED				
THU				
FRI				
SAT				
SUN				

Shopping list

_________________ _________________

_________________ _________________

_________________ _________________

Notes:

Weekly
Meal Plan

Week: _______________

	BREAKFAST	LUNCH	DINNER	SNACKS
MON				
TUE				
WED				
THU				
FRI				
SAT				
SUN				

Shopping list

_____________ _____________

_____________ _____________

_____________ _____________

Notes:

Weekly
Meal Plan

Week: ______________

	BREAKFAST	LUNCH	DINNER	SNACKS
MON				
TUE				
WED				
THU				
FRI				
SAT				
SUN				

Shopping list

_______________ _______________

_______________ _______________

_______________ _______________

Notes:

Weekly
Meal Plan

Week:________________

	BREAKFAST	LUNCH	DINNER	SNACKS
MON				
TUE				
WED				
THU				
FRI				
SAT				
SUN				

Shopping list

___________   ___________

___________   ___________

___________   ___________

Notes:

Weekly
Meal Plan

Week: ______________

	BREAKFAST	LUNCH	DINNER	SNACKS
MON				
TUE				
WED				
THU				
FRI				
SAT				
SUN				

Shopping list

______________ ______________

______________ ______________

______________ ______________

Notes: